Manual of Aphasia Therapy

MW01057041

Manual of
Aphasia Therapy

Nancy Helm-Estabrooks, Sc.D.
Martin L. Albert, M.D.

Department of Neurology
Aphasia Research Center
Boston University School of Medicine
and
Boston Veterans Administration Medical Center

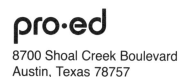

8700 Shoal Creek Boulevard
Austin, Texas 78757

Printed in the United States of America

Library of Congress Cataloging-in-Publication Data

Helm-Estabrooks, Nancy, 1940–
    Manual of aphasia therapy / Nancy Helm-Estabrooks, Martin L.
Albert.
      p.   cm.
    Includes bibliographical references.
    ISBN 0-89079-404-9
    1. Aphasia—Treatment—Handbooks, manuals, etc. I. Albert,
Martin L., 1939- . II. Title.
    [DNLM: 1. Aphasia—diagnosis. 2. Aphasia—therapy.
WL 340.5   H478m]
RC425.H45   1991
616.85′52061—dc20
DNLM/DLC
for Library of Congress   90–5630
                                         CIP

pro·ed

8700 Shoal Creek Boulevard
Austin, Texas 78757

4 5 6 7 8 9 10   97 96 95 94 93

Contents

Preface

For over 18 years we have worked together within the settings of a hospital ward for aphasia patients, an aphasia research center, and a medical school. One of us is a speech and language pathologist and the other a neurologist, but we both are clinicians, researchers, and teachers. As such, we examine and treat patients, develop and test experimental rehabilitation methods, and train students in our respective fields. In writing this manual we have called upon our combined experience. We have tried to create a book that serves as a candid reflection of our day-to-day concerns with aphasia. In particular, we wanted to describe our approach to clinical problem solving, starting with the language-impaired patient and moving through a series of logical steps to the development of an aphasia rehabilitation program shaped to the needs of the individual patient. This book is written in the language and style that we use on our daily bedside rounds, in our teaching conferences, and with our research colleagues.

The process of aphasia rehabilitation begins with an understanding of the neuroanatomy of language and the neuropathology of aphasia (chapters 1 and 2). The system we use for classifying aphasia, often called "the Boston aphasia classification system," has been simplified in this manual with our diagrammatic representation of an aphasia taxonomy "tree" (chapter 3).

An accurate and thorough diagnosis of aphasia requires a multidisciplinary approach, beginning with the neurologic examination (chapter 4) that incorporates ancillary neurodiagnostic techniques (chapter 5). Because many patients with aphasia due to stroke have specific medical or neurologic illnesses that may affect their response to treatment, a discussion of these possibilities is presented in chapter 6. We believe that successful aphasia rehabilitation programs are built on a patient's strengths, or islands of preserved abilities, in the areas of cognition, memory, and verbal and nonverbal communication. A full identification of these strengths requires a neuropsychologic examination, an aphasia examination, and an apraxia examination (chapters 7, 8, and 9). We are grateful to our colleague, Roberta Gallagher, Boston University Aphasia Research Center, for authoring our chapter on "the process approach" to the neuropsychologic examination.

The process approach to evaluation of the aphasic patient focuses not simply on final scores but on the exact nature of the patient's response as he or she tries to perform correctly to any stimulus or task. Chapter 10 describes how the process approach to the examination of aphasia can be used to generate effective treatment programs. The next issue, then, is the measurement of aphasia treatment effects, which we address in chapter 11.

Our chapters on specific approaches to aphasia rehabilitation describe the methods that we and our colleagues have developed at the Aphasia Research Center, an interdisciplinary program within the Department of Neurology of Boston University School of Medicine and the Boston Veterans Administration Medical Center. These include two nonvocal programs: Visual Action Therapy and "Back to the Drawing Board" (chapters 12 and 13); four verbal output programs: Voluntary Control of Involuntary Utterances, Melodic Intonation Therapy, Syntax Stimulation, and Treatment for Aphasic Perseveration (chapters 14–17); one program for treatment of auditory comprehension deficits in Wernicke's aphasia (chapter 18); and pharmacotherapy for aphasia (chapter 19). The final chapters of this manual discuss the psychological, neuropsychiatric, legal, and social impact of aphasia on the patient and family (chapters 20 and 21).

Our success depends upon the help, guidance, support, cooperation, and advice of our patients, their families, and our co-workers. Although the material presented in this manual represents our personal approach to aphasia rehabilitation, we have been greatly influenced by our many friends and colleagues, including Frank Benson, Howard Gardner, Loraine Obler, Edgar Zurif, Patricia Fitzpatrick, Sheila Blumstein, Laird Cermak, Marlene Oscar-Berman, Margaret Naeser, and the many other participants in Aphasia Research Center activity over the years. In particular, we would like to express special and deep appreciation to Harold Goodglass and Edith Kaplan, and, in memoriam, to Norman Geschwind.

We also wish to acknowledge several people who helped bring this book to fruition. First and foremost we thank Suzanne Ruscitti, who logged hundreds of hours at her word processor typing numerous versions of each chapter from the roughest draft to the finished product. John Dyke drew the excellent illustrations from the bits and pieces we handed him.

Marjorie Nicholas, Alan Mandell, Patricia Fitzpatrick, and Suzanne Miller read drafts and offered suggestions for improvement. Throughout the development, writing, and publication process our editor, Marie Linvill, kept us goal directed while maintaining her own equanimity.

Ours has been a rewarding, and always instructive, experience in treating aphasia patients. We hope this manual conveys the positive attitude we have developed in our daily confrontation with aphasia.

Section One
Foundations of Aphasia Rehabilitation

Neuroanatomy of Language

An introduction to the study of aphasia must first consider the neural basis of language, that is, the normal apparatus. However, a comprehensive map of brain-language relationships is far from fully developed, and new techniques of brain imaging have considerably modified classical teachings. Nevertheless, much of what had been taught in the past retains current clinical validity, such as that lesions in the "zone of language" in the left hemisphere of most right-handed people usually will produce aphasia. However, many additional regions of the brain are known to contribute to language function, including right hemispheric and subcortical structures. This chapter and those that follow will demonstrate that knowledge of the widely distributed anatomical substrate for language can be exploited for development of creative new approaches to aphasia therapy.

To understand the anatomy of language, one should have a general understanding of neuroanatomy. From the effector organ (e.g., muscle) inward, the following components of the nervous system should be considered: peripheral nerves, spinal cord, brain stem, cerebellum, subcortical nuclear structures (subcortical gray matter), subcortical white matter (association pathways, commissures, corpus callosum), and cortex. At the same time, one must have a picture of how these various anatomical systems are organized regionally (e.g., limbic system, frontal lobe, temporal lobe, etc.).

Specific neuroanatomical structures *never* function in complete isolation from other parts of the brain. All complex cognitive skills, such as language, arise from the interaction of multiple anatomical regions, that is, overlapping and interconnected neural networks widely distributed throughout the brain, carrying out their specific neural functions both sequentially and in parallel. The concept of **parallel distributed processing (PDP)**, popular in contemporary cognitive science, provides a useful metaphor for the understanding of higher cortical functions in humans. The simplest language task depends on a complex interaction of the reticular activating system, subcortical nuclear structures, right hemisphere, subcortical white matter, and left-hemispheric "zone of language."

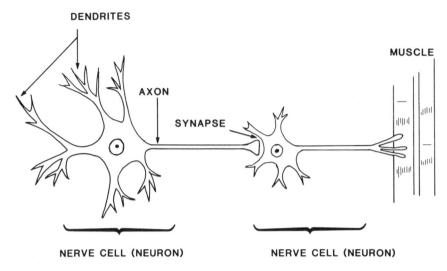

FIG. 1.1. Neurons

I. Neuroanatomical Structures

A. Basic Components

Nerve cells (neurons) comprise the basic elements, the build-ing blocks, of the nervous system. Each neuron consists of a cell body and branching processes called nerve fibers. **Dendrites** are short nerve fibers that receive electrochemical impulses and transport these impulses toward the cell body. An **axon** is a long nerve fiber that generally transports impulses away from the cell body (see Fig. 1.1).

Neural transmission (Fig. 1.2) refers to the transfer of elec-trochemical impulses (or "information") from one neuron to another. **Neurotransmitters** are chemical substances, such as dopamine or acetylcholine, that may be transferred from one neuron to another, or that may facilitate or interfere with neu-ral transmission. Neural transmission takes place at a **syn-apse** or junction between two neurons. Often the axon of one neuron connects with the dendrites of another neuron. In such a transmission pathway, the **afferent fiber** is the one carrying a neural impulse toward the cell body, while the **efferent fiber** is the one carrying the impulse away from a cell body.

Neurons (cell body and fibers) generally are organized in clus-ters. A cluster of nerve cell bodies located within the brain or

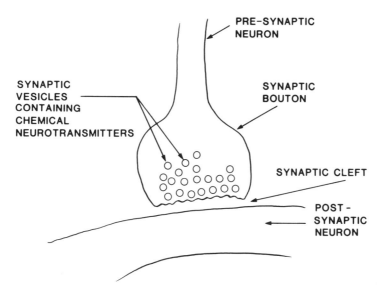

FIG. 1.2. Chemical synaptic neurotransmission. Chemical neurotransmitters are released from synaptic vesicles in the presynaptic neuron, pass across the synaptic cleft, and excite or inhibit the postsynaptic neuron.

spinal cord is called a **nucleus**. A cluster of nerve cell bodies located outside the brain and spinal cord is called a **ganglion**. A cluster of nerve fibers within the brain or spinal cord that has a common origin and common final end point may be called a **tract, column, commissure, fasciculus,** or **pathway. Gray matter** refers to regions of the brain or spinal cord containing clusters of nerve cell bodies. In a postmortem examination of the brain, clusters of nerve cell bodies appear gray, in contrast with collections of white or cream-colored nerve fibers, which are called **white matter.** The cerebral cortex consists of layers of nerve cells, appears gray in color, and is included with cerebral nuclei as the gray matter of the brain.

B. Peripheral Nerves

The **peripheral nervous system** consists of cranial nerves (e.g., olfactory, optic, facial, auditory) and spinal nerves. Nerves may be motor (innervating effector organs such as voluntary and involuntary muscles) or sensory. Sensory fibers receive stimuli from receptor organs (e.g., touch, pressure, pain, heat, cold) and transmit information centrally. Collections of nerve fibers outside the spinal cord are variously called **nerves, nerve roots,** or **nerve trunks**.

C. Central Nervous System

The central nervous system includes the brain (gray and white matter of the cerebral hemispheres, brain stem, and cerebellum) and spinal cord. The brain, about the size of a small grapefruit, weighs about 1,250 grams and is composed of an estimated 15 billion neurons plus supporting cells.

D. Spinal Cord

The spinal cord travels through the vertebral column carrying neural impulses from the periphery to the brain for further analysis and from the brain to the periphery to produce responses. Spinal nerves appear in pairs, one on each side of the cord. There are 31 of these pairs: 8 cervical, 12 thoracic, 5 lumbar, 5 sacral, and 1 coccygeal.

E. Brain Stem

The brain stem is divided into three segments: medulla, pons, and midbrain. The **medulla oblongata**, or **medulla**, is the continuation of the spinal cord through the base of the skull. This portion of the brain stem contains nuclei for the cranial nerves responsible for movements of the tongue, orpharynx, larynx, and diaphragm. Cough and gag reflexes also are mediated at this level of the brain.

The **pons** is continuous with the medulla, and the **midbrain** is continuous with the pons. These segments of the brain contain cranial nerve nuclei for eye movements, facial expression, facial sensation, and hearing.

F. Cerebellum

The cerebellum sits like a roof over the brain stem and is composed of a surface layer of gray matter and an inner core of white matter and cerebellar nuclei. The cerebellum consists of two large lateral masses, the **cerebellar hemispheres** (to be distinguished from the cerebral hemispheres) and a narrow midline portion, the **vermis**. The cerebellum is responsible for integrating or coordinating muscle groups throughout the body. To function normally, motor activity must flow with a smooth, regular, well-timed, well-coordinated rhythm. The cerebellum maintains this rhythm. Abnormalities of cerebellar function

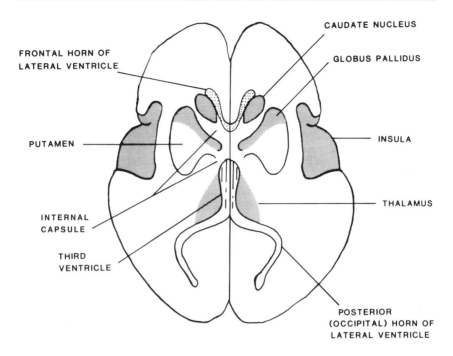

FIG. 1.3. Subcortical structures, horizontal view

may affect the muscles of the glossopharyngeal apparatus, producing speech disorders such as **dysarthria** or **ataxia**.

G. Subcortical Gray Matter

Deep within the cerebral hemispheres are several collections of nerve cell bodies that comprise the subcortical gray matter, serving a variety of sensory, motor, and integrative functions. These structures (see Fig. 1.3) include the **diencephalon** and the **basal ganglia**. The diencephalon consists primarily of the **thalamus** and **hypothalamus** and their connections. The basal ganglia consist primarily of the **caudate nucleus**, **putamen**, **globus pallidus**, and **amygdala**.

The **thalamus**, long known as a major way station along the route from peripheral sensation to cortical association areas, serves at least two additional functions, both important for language. One of these functions has to do with focusing attention. Attentional mechanisms involve considerable processing of stimuli (incoming stimuli must be selected, filtered, directed to the correct location, etc.), and apparently the thalamus, at least in part, plays this role. Segments of the thalamus also participate in processes of memory. Because normal language function depends on attentional and mnestic activity, not surprisingly lesions of the thalamus have been implicated in syndromes of aphasia. Thalamic lesions, especially in the left hemisphere, often are linked to fluctuating attention and problems with verbal memory.

While the thalamus is the major subcortical nuclear structure responsible for sensory transmission and sensory integration, the caudate, putamen, and globus pallidus govern motor control and motor integration. The **pyramidal system** of the motor cortex (see section II.A. "Frontal Lobes") controls voluntary movements in the body. Execution of voluntary motor activity is regulated, modulated, modified, speeded up or slowed down, and increased or decreased in amplitude by the **extrapyramidal system**. The extrapyramidal system includes, in addition to other structures, the caudate, putamen, and globus pallidus. Damage to these structures or their major connections can cause abnormalities of speed, for example, bradykinesia (slowness of movement) may be seen in Parkinson's disease, a disorder of basal ganglia and their connections; and involuntary movements are seen in Huntington's disease, a degenerative disorder starting in the caudate.

Lesions of basal ganglia have been linked to symptoms found within aphasic syndromes. Small bilateral lesions of the basal ganglia are often the cause of hypophonic speech. Dysarthria may result from damage to basal ganglia; if the damage is unilateral, the dysarthria is usually transient. Nonfluent and fluent aphasias (see chapter 3) as well as global aphasia can result from left-hemispheric lesions in the region of the basal ganglia. It has not been ascertained whether these subcortical aphasic syndromes result from damage to subcortical nuclei (gray matter), pathways (white matter), or both.

H. Subcortical White Matter

Clusters or layers of nerve cell bodies within the brain (nuclei, gray matter) are responsible for organizing, integrating, analyzing, and synthesizing neural impulses. As previously asserted, however, no region of the brain functions in complete isolation from others. Gray matter clusters are preferentially connected to other gray matter clusters by means of nerve fiber pathways, the white matter. Selected groups of nerve cell bodies together with their interconnecting nerve fiber pathways are called **neural networks**. Complex cognitive functions arise from neurotransmission within and across multiple, widely distributed neural networks. It follows that lesions anywhere within a single neural network, whether in the gray matter cluster or in the white matter transmission pathway, may interfere with the cognitive function and produce a neurobehavioral syndrome such as aphasia. It follows equally that knowledge of which neural networks are disrupted *and which neural networks are spared* may lead to development of treatment approaches that utilize spared or only partially impaired systems.

Among the white matter pathways of most interest to the specialist in aphasia are the **corpus callosum**, the **cortico-cortical association fibers**, and the **cortico-subcortical connections**.

The two cerebral hemispheres are separated by a dividing space (the **median longitudinal fissure**), at the base of which is a broad, thick band of white matter (the corpus callosum) that joins the two hemispheres. Divided into three segments (genu, rostrum, and splenium), the corpus callosum links corresponding regions of the two hemispheres. Damage to one or another segment of the corpus callosum will interrupt the transfer of information from one hemisphere to another and may result in the appearance of abnormalities of cognitive function, such as disorders of reading, naming, or voluntary control of movement. Because these neurobehavioral syndromes result from the disconnection of one part of the brain from another, they are often called **disconnection syndromes**.

Cortico-cortical association fibers connect different regions of the cortex to each other. In his 1965 paper "Disconnexion Syndromes in Animals and Man," Norman Geschwind provided a speculative explanation of the process of naming based in large part on the availability in the human brain of cortico-cortical association fibers. Of particular interest for the anatomy of language are the **superior longitudinal fasciculus**, a white matter pathway connecting posterior cortical sensory association areas with frontal motor association areas, and the **arcuate fasciculus**, a smaller bundle of nerve fibers arching from the auditory association area in the temporal lobe (Wernicke's area) and joining the superior longitudinal fasciculus, eventually making its way to the frontal motor association cortex

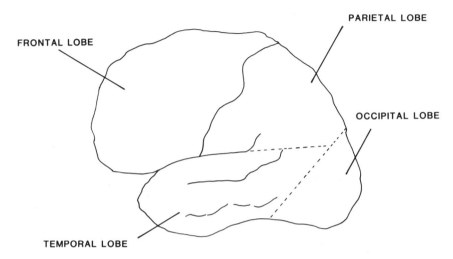

FIG. 1.4. Brain, lateral view, left hemisphere, lobes

for the muscles of the glossopharyngeal apparatus (Broca's area). Several lesions in the brain can produce the aphasic feature of impaired repetition of speech; one of these lesions is in the arcuate fasciculus.

New brain imaging techniques have revealed the importance of subcortical structures in language. It seems that cortico-subcortical white matter pathways may be equally important. Because cortical gray matter and subcortical nuclei are connected by white matter pathways into neural networks that subserve language function, lesions in these white matter pathways may lead to aphasic phenomena.

I. Cortex

The outermost surface of the brain is covered by sheets of nerve cells (gray matter) called the **cerebral cortex**. The surface of each hemisphere appears as a convoluted mass of ridges and furrows; the eminences on these ridges are called **gyri**, the grooves **sulci**. Two large grooves (fissures) divide the brain into four sections or lobes (see Fig. 1.4) Each of the four major lobes of the brain is responsible for primary functions and higher order secondary functions, the so-called "higher cortical functions." The **sylvian (or lateral) fissure** is a large furrow beginning on the base of the brain and extending laterally upward. The **temporal lobe** is located beside and below the sylvian fis-

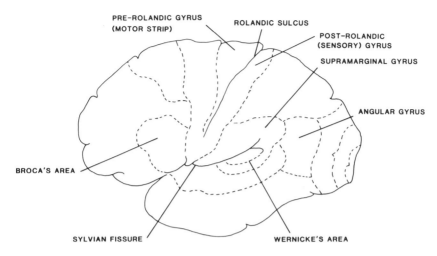

FIG. 1.5. Brain, lateral view, left hemisphere, gyri and sulci

sure. The **fissure of Rolando (central sulcus)** is a large furrow running downward and forward from the top of the brain just past its midpoint almost to the sylvian fissure. In front of the fissure of Rolando is the **frontal lobe.** The **parietal lobe** sits behind the fissure of Rolando and above the sylvian fissure, extending back to about 2 inches from the posterior part of the brain. The **occipital lobe** occupies the posterior 2 inches. The cerebral cortex is responsible for high order analysis, integration, and synthesis of neural impulses arriving from the periphery. Figs. 1.5, 1.6, and 1.7 further detail the various structures of the brain.

II. Regional Organization

A. Frontal Lobes

The primary function of the frontal lobes is voluntary control of movement throughout the body. Within the frontal lobe, just in front of the central sulcus, is a gyrus called the **motor strip**. Just behind the central sulcus is a gyrus called the **sensory strip** (located in the parietal lobe). These two gyri, known as the **sensorimotor cortex**, work together to control willed movements on the side of the body opposite the hemisphere in question (left hemisphere, right side of body). The motor strip sends its neural messages to the muscles via a set of pathways and nuclei cumulatively called the **pyramidal system**. Voluntary

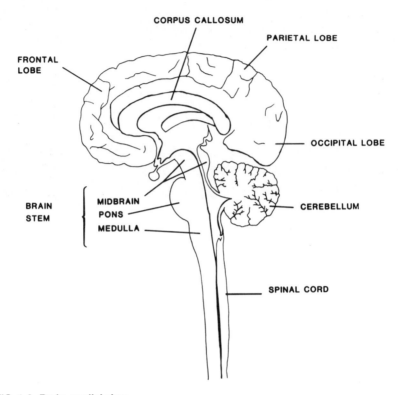

FIG. 1.6. Brain, medial view

control of motor behavior is modulated by the **extrapyramidal system**, which is a complex neural network comprising the premotor frontal cortex, subcortical gray matter, cerebellum, and vestibular system. Lesions in pyramidal or extrapyramidal systems can provoke speech or language disorders, as will be discussed in subsequent chapters.

Anterior to the motor strip is a portion of frontal lobe called the **supplementary motor cortex**. This region of the brain may play a critical role for language, as it seems partially responsible for initiation of motor activity. The ability to initiate spontaneous utterances is impaired by lesions in this region or in the white matter pathways descending from this area to subcortical motor structures.

The **frontal premotor association cortex** is thought to be responsible for synthesizing sensory stimuli coming from throughout

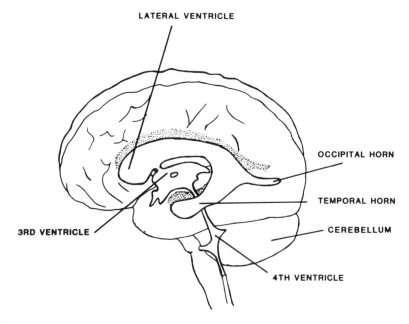

FIG. 1.7. Ventricles of the brain

the brain and coordinating them with plans for action. Thus, the frontal lobe apparently mediates abstract thinking, problem solving, and judgment. Damage to this portion of the brain may cause behavioral and personality changes, including impaired judgment, poor strategic planning, and impaired insight, all of which are important, of course, for normal language function.

B. Temporal Lobes

The primary function of the temporal lobes is hearing. Nerve fibers travel from the cranial auditory nerves through the brainstem and thalamus to the **auditory cortex** in the temporal lobe, making many intermediate connections along the way. Neural impulses from peripheral and central auditory pathways then undergo elaboration and analysis in the auditory association area, located in the posterior portion of the **superior temporal gyrus (Wernicke's area)**.

This region is responsible for developing the analysis of auditory stimuli to the point of comprehension. This task is carried out by means of multiple cortico-cortical associations, linking auditory stimuli with those from other sensory systems. Important for this function are memory systems organized as neural networks within temporal lobes and subcortical gray and white matter structures.

C. Parietal Lobes

The primary function of the parietal lobes is perception and elaboration of somesthetic sensations (bodily awareness sensations, including touch, pressure, and position in space). As with motor control in the frontal lobes, somesthesis is organized in the hemisphere opposite the side of the body involved (e.g., left side of body, right hemisphere). Somesthetic sensations reach the **post-central gyrus** (the first gyrus in the parietal lobe just past the central sulcus), also called the **sensory strip**.

These stimuli travel by means of short association fibers to the **secondary sensory association regions,** located more posteriorly in the parietal lobe. Here the somesthetic sensations are analyzed, elaborated, and connected with multiple stimuli arriving from other parts of the brain. Eventually, with second- and third-order processing of neural stimuli, an image of one's own body and its position in space emerges. Damage to this part of the brain can produce not only a loss of sensation of touch but also impaired recognition of own's own body (asomatognosia) and a loss of the ability to appreciate spatial concepts.

D. Occipital Lobes

The primary function of the occipital lobes is vision. The retina of the eye receives visual stimuli and then transmits them via the optic nerve and the thalamus to the **primary visual cortex** in the occipital lobe. Here the neural impulses are perceived as meaningless flashes of light. To be understood in a meaningful way, the neural information within the visual system must be further analyzed, elaborated, and connected with stimuli from other parts of the brain and from memory systems as well. This higher order analysis takes place in the **visual association cortex**, which extends beyond the primary visual area on the medial and lateral surfaces of the occipital lobe.

E. Limbic System

The limbic system (Fig. 1.8) is a complex network of cortical and subcortical (gray and white matter) structures that medi-

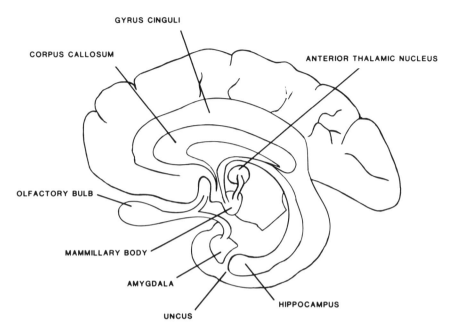

GYRUS CINGULI

CORPUS CALLOSUM

ANTERIOR THALAMIC NUCLEUS

OLFACTORY BULB

MAMMILLARY BODY

AMYGDALA

UNCUS

HIPPOCAMPUS

FIG. 1.8. Limbic system

ates emotion. Major elements of the limbic system include the **uncus** (a portion of the olfactory system), the **para-hippocampal gyrus**, the **hippocampus** (a portion of the memory system within the temporal lobes), the **fornix** (a major association pathway), the **mammillary bodies** (in the thalamic region), the **mammillo-thalamic tract**, and the **cingulate gyrus** (which lies over the corpus callosum). Closely linked to the limbic system are the hypothalamus, amygdala, and frontal association cortex.

Memories, the desire to produce language, feelings, and the emotional coloring of thought are all mediated by the limbic system. Anatomical systems necessary for cognitive functions, such as language, spatial concepts, understanding of meaning in life, and so forth are all intimately linked to the limbic system. Thus, aphasia therapy programs may be developed that exploit affective or limbic aspects of language.

F. "Zone of Language"

The zone of language was defined by Dejerine in the early 1900s as that region of the left hemisphere responsible for language (see Fig. 1.9). Located within the distribution of the mid-

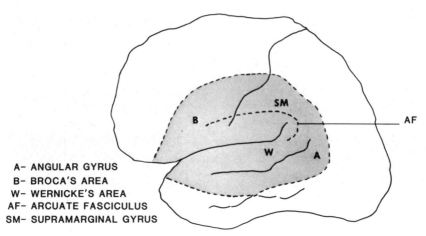

A- ANGULAR GYRUS
B- BROCA'S AREA
W- WERNICKE'S AREA
AF- ARCUATE FASCICULUS
SM- SUPRAMARGINAL GYRUS

FIG. 1.9. "Zone of language"

dle cerebral artery, the zone of language surrounds the sylvian fissure on the lateral surface of the hemisphere, incorporating portions of the frontal, parietal, and temporal lobes. Anteriorly the zone extends to Broca's area (in the premotor region of the frontal lobe adjacent to the portion of the motor strip responsible for the muscles of the glossopharyngeal apparatus). Posteriorly it extends to Wernicke's area (the auditory association cortex in the posterior portion of the superior temporal gyrus). Connecting Wernicke's area and Broca's area are subcortical white matter pathways, including the arcuate fasciculus and superior longitudinal fasciculus. These white matter pathways pass through the angular gyrus and supramarginal gyrus at the posterior rim of the sylvian fissure, where temporal and parietal lobes come together. These gyri are association areas where many neural interconnections from all over the brain occur. As described in chapter 2, lesions in different parts of the zone of language may produce different aphasia syndromes.

The zone of language should not be considered a "center" for language (i.e., a region of the brain where language is located). Rather, it should be regarded as a critical component of several overlapping neural networks, widely distributed throughout the brain, whose total combined activity has the effect of producing language as we know it.

Selected Readings

Brodal, A. (1981). *Neurological anatomy* (3rd ed.). New York: Oxford University Press.

Geschwind, N. (1965). Disconnexion syndromes in animals and man. *Brain, 88,* 237–294, 585–644.

Nauta, W.J.H., & Feirtag, M. (1986). *Fundamental neuroanatomy.* New York: W.H. Freeman.

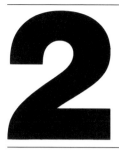

Neuropathology of Aphasia

The traditional localizationist approach to aphasia, based on clinico-pathological studies, relies on neuroanatomic conceptions developed in the 19th century by such clinicians as Broca, Wernicke, and Lichtheim and extended in the 20th century by neuroscientists such as Dejerine and Geschwind. This classical approach is still the most popular and has undeniable clinical relevance.

However, newer insights into brain-language relations have resulted from neuroimaging studies in normal and aphasic subjects. Contemporary cognitive neuroscience has rediscovered old anti-localizationist views, such as those of Marie, Head, Goldstein, Bay, and Lashley, which declare the localizationist views outmoded and wrong. These arguments, although often unnecessarily antagonistic, arise from important neuroscientific data and are potentially useful for developing new ideas in aphasia therapy.

Our own conception of the anatomy of language and neuropathology of aphasia is based on a model that attempts to account for three different sets of neurological evidence, supporting the concurrent existence of (a) widely distributed, (b) regional, and (c) highly localized neural correlates of language. This conception will be reviewed briefly at the end of this chapter.

I. Traditional Localizationist Approaches

Cerebral dominance for language is a concept of brain-language relationships that asserts, in its extreme form, that one hemisphere (major, leading, or dominant) contains the neural structures responsible for language, while the other hemisphere (minor, following, or subdominant) does not contribute to language. In this form the concept is clearly incorrect. A less extreme version of the same basic idea states that the dominant hemisphere contains more of whatever it is that is important for language, while the other hemisphere contains less. More recent notions of cerebral dominance accept the fact that both hemispheres contribute varying degrees of different components of language function. Nevertheless, if one hemisphere is damaged and a person is rendered aphasic, that hemisphere is considered the language-dominant hemisphere.

It is generally agreed that more than 99% of right-handers have left-hemispheric dominance for language. With the evolution of concepts of cerebral dominance, however, has come acceptance of the fact that even in right-handers the right hemisphere contributes to language function. Thus, it is widely recognized that the right hemisphere contributes to prosodic and pragmatic aspects of language. This fact can be quite important for language rehabilitation.

As for left-handers, the situation is less certain. The degree to which left-handers have right, left, or bilateral hemispheric dominance for language is not known. Evidence supports the contention that approximately 70% of left-handers may have left-hemispheric dominance for language, while the other 30% may have bilateral dominance. It is possible that brain-language relations for all left-handers are different from those for right-handers.

According to the classical view, the zone of language in the left hemisphere contains cortical centers that support specific language functions, the centers being interconnected. A lesion in any of these centers or in the connections between any two centers will produce a characteristic and predictable form of aphasia. This classical view has persisted in a relatively unmodified form for more than a century. The simple reason for the persistence of this localizationist-connectionist model, despite continuous challenge, is that it has been supported consistently by clinicopathological correlations.

In considering clinicopathological correlations for the major syndromes of aphasia, one must exercise a measure of caution. Even strict localizationists concede that not all aphasia syndromes can be explained by classical models. Approximately 80% of aphasia syndromes conform roughly to this anatomoclinical scheme; the remaining 20% may be explained by individual differences in brain structure or other factors. A lesion in one part of the brain may produce different syndromes in different patients; a lesion in widely varying parts of the brain may occasionally produce a similar syndrome in different patients. Among the factors influencing variability is lesion etiology. A brain tumor or a patch of focal encephalitis may affect local brain tissue differently than a stroke, for

TABLE 2.1
Aphasia Localization

Aphasia type	Lesion location
Broca's	Lateral frontal, suprasylvian, prerolandic, extending into adjacent subcortical periventricular white matter
Wernicke's	Posterior third of superior temporal gyrus
Conduction	White matter pathways under supramarginal gyrus
Anomic	Augular gyrus; second temporal gyrus
Transcortical motor	Anterior frontal paramedian; anterior and superior to Broca's area
Transcortical sensory	Posterior parieto-temporal, sparing Wernicke's area
Global	Large perisylvian, extending deep into subjacent white matter
Subcortical	1. Thalamic 2. Caudate, putamen, and/or internal capsule

example. Age, handedness, prior brain damage, the presence of seizures, depression, or other medical or psychiatric disorders all may influence brain-behavior relations. An overview of lesion locations and the resulting type of aphasia is presented in Table 2.1.

A. Broca's Aphasia

The lesion most commonly associated with Broca's aphasia is large and involves the left lateral frontal, prerolandic, suprasylvian region (Broca's area) extending necessarily into the periventricular white matter deep to Broca's area. This lesion is in the territory of the superior division of the middle cerebral artery and often extends posteriorly to include the parietal lobe (see Figs. 2.1 and 2.2). A lesion *limited* to Broca's area (the foot of the inferior frontal gyrus), however, does not produce Broca's aphasia. Such a lesion produces mild dysprosody and mild agraphia, occasionally accompanied by word-finding pauses and mild dysarthria.

Over the years debate has ensued about whether the inferior prerolandic motor strip (i.e., the motor cortex region responsible for the control of the muscles of the glossopharyngeal apparatus) must be included in the lesion producing Broca's aphasia. Part of the debate is based on the evidence that a lesion limited to this region may be responsible for the syndrome of

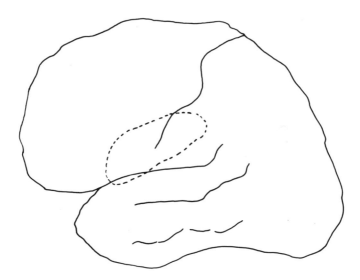

FIG. 2.1. Broca's aphasia, lateral view

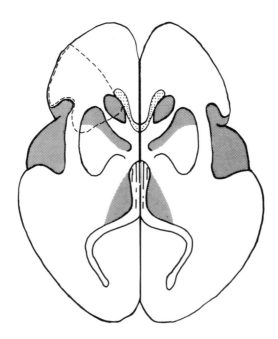

FIG. 2.2. Broca's aphasia, horizontal view

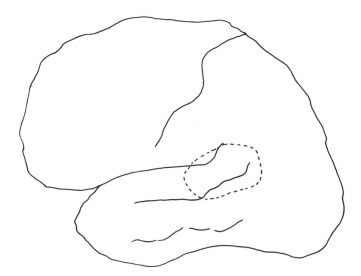

FIG. 2.3. Wernicke's aphasia, lateral view

aphemia (pure word dumbness, pure motor aphasia). Aphemia is not truly an aphasic syndrome, but rather an isolated loss of the ability to articulate words, without a loss of the ability to write or to comprehend spoken or written language.

B. Wernicke's Aphasia

Wernicke's aphasia is produced by lesions in the posterior third of the superior temporal gyrus (Wernicke's area), in the distribution of the inferior division of the middle cerebral artery (see Figs. 2.3 and 2.4). At least two forms of this aphasia have been defined by anatomical locus of lesion. A primarily temporal lesion produces a word deaf variant in which reading may be relatively less affected; patients have great difficulty comprehending individual isolated words but can more easily understand words in context. If the lesion extends posteriorly, visual connections are disrupted; the patient will have more difficulty understanding written language and language in context but relatively less difficulty with isolated words.

C. Conduction Aphasia

A lesion in the white matter pathways (arcuate fasciculus, superior longitudinal fasciculus) connecting Wernicke's area to Broca's area may produce conduction aphasia (see Figs. 2.5 and

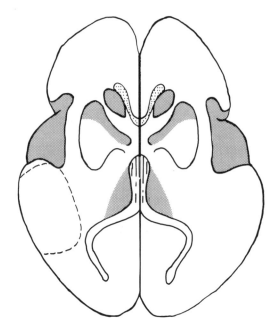

FIG. 2.4. Wernicke's aphasia, horizontal view

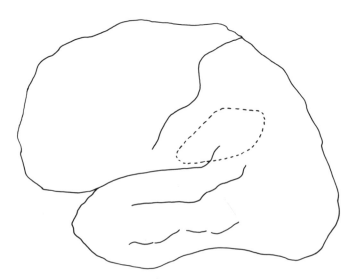

FIG. 2.5. Conduction aphasia, lateral view

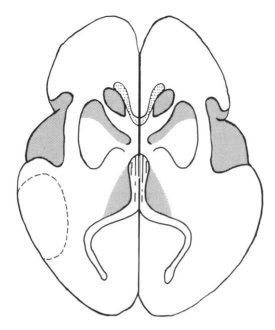

FIG. 2.6. Conduction aphasia, horizontal view

2.6). This lesion generally is located in the region of the supra-marginal gyrus or inferior parietal lobule. Rarely, lesions limited to Wernicke's area may produce a true conduction aphasia, with no defect in auditory comprehension.

D. Anomic Aphasia

On the one hand, anomia is the least useful localizing sign in aphasia because any lesion in or near the zone of language can produce anomia. Indeed, virtually every aphasic syndrome contains an anomic component. On the other hand, lesions of the angular gyrus often produce anomic aphasia in conjunction with other neurobehavioral phenomena, and anomic aphasias also have been produced selectively by lesions of the second temporal gyrus. Fig. 2.7 identifies the typical lesion sites that produce anomic aphasia. One should also be aware that other common forms of aphasia often evolve to a syndrome of primarily anomic aphasia in the process of recovery.

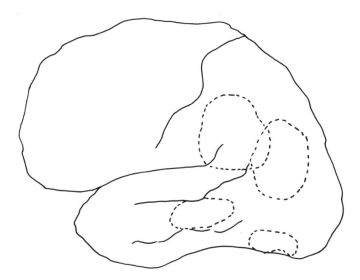

FIG. 2.7. Anomic aphasia, lateral view

E. Transcortical Motor Aphasia

An anteriorly (frontally) located lesion that interrupts the link between supplementary motor cortex and Broca's area, but spares Broca's area, will produce a transcortical motor aphasia. Such a lesion may be in more than one location: in the supplementary motor cortex itself, in white matter pathways underneath the supplementary motor area, or in the left frontal lobe, anterior and superior to Broca's area (see Fig. 2.8). These lesions are caused by disruption of flow either in the anterior cerebral artery or in the anterior-most penetrating branches of the middle cerebral artery. Infarction in the border-zone territory between anterior and middle cerebral arteries seems to be a common cause.

F. Transcortical Sensory Aphasia

Posterior lesions in the border zone between the middle and posterior cerebral arteries, in parietotemporal regions sparing Wernicke's area, can cause transcortical sensory aphasia (see Fig. 2.9). Looking carefully at this syndrome one may be struck by the frequency of its association with bilateral lesions (in border-zone territory). Interestingly, transcortical sensory aphasia is one of the common forms of aphasia seen in Alz-

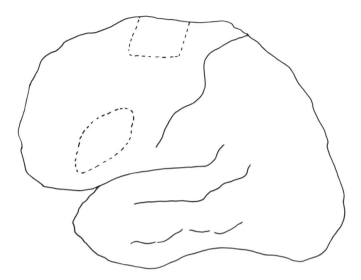

FIG. 2.8. Transcortical motor aphasia, lateral view

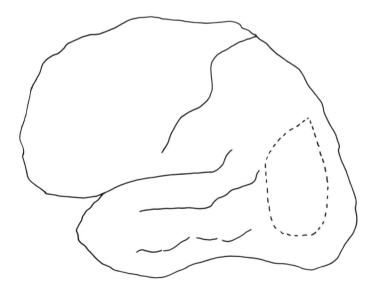

FIG. 2.9. Transcortical sensory aphasia, lateral view

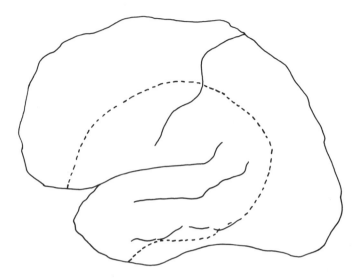

FIG. 2.10. Global aphasia, lateral view

heimer's disease, a disease with bilateral posterior association cortex lesions.

G. Global Aphasia

Infarction in the territory of both divisions of the middle cerebral artery produces global aphasia. Destruction of brain tissue occurs in large portions of the left fronto-parieto-temporal zone of language, extending from Broca's area to Wernicke's area to the angular gyrus region and deep into subjacent white matter (see Figs. 2.10 and 2.11). The term **global aphasia** implies a severe language defect across all language modalities; milder versions are called **mixed aphasias**.

H. Subcortical Aphasias

Precise clinicopathological correlates have not been defined yet for the subcortical aphasias. The story is still unfolding, and a complete systematization of clinical syndrome and anatomical locus of lesion remains to be developed. In broad terms, two major varieties of subcortical aphasia can be identified. In one form, regions of the basal ganglia (especially the caudate and putamen) and/or adjacent regions of the internal capsule (especially the anterior limb) have been implicated (Fig. 2.12). In the

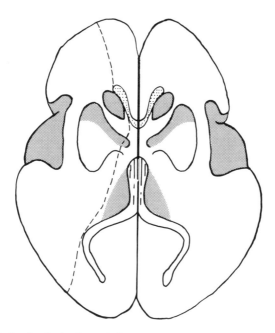

FIG. 2.11. **Global aphasia, horizontal view**

other, the lesions are located in the left (dominant) thalamus, particularly the pulvinar (Fig. 2.13).

I. Cerebrovascular System and Aphasia

A major cerebrovascular distinction can be drawn between disorders of oral language and those of written language. When brain damage is vascular in cause and the language problem affects written language only, the lesion is usually in the distribution of the posterior cerebral artery. When the language problem is exclusively oral, the lesion is usually in the distribution of the middle cerebral artery. When both spoken and written language are affected, the lesion is usually in the distribution of the internal carotid artery.

The "zone of language" falls within the territory of the middle cerebral artery, which has an inferior and a superior division. Infarction in the respective branches of the middle cerebral artery produces damage to the inferior or superior bank of the sylvian fissure and generally causes aphasia with repeti-

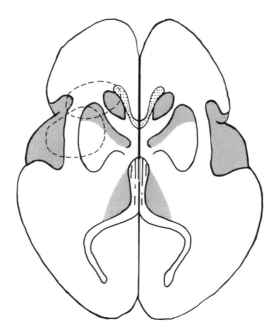

FIG. 2.12. Anterior subcortical aphasia, horizontal view

tion defect (Broca's, Wernicke's, conduction aphasia). When a patient displays an aphasic syndrome with preserved ability to repeat, the lesion usually has spared the cortical zone of language but involved cortical or subcortical areas bordering the language zone (transcortical aphasias; subcortical aphasias). These border-zone lesions may be secondary to occlusion of the internal carotid artery. Fig. 2.14 details the system of blood supply to the zone of language.

II. Contemporary Views of Brain-Language Relations

The study of the neurological basis of language has been revolutionized in the past 20 years by the development of noninvasive in vivo neuroimaging techniques. These new diagnostic procedures have made it possible to test neurolinguistic theories directly by evaluating brain function in both the damaged and the undamaged portions of the brain.

Current theory in aphasia rejects the notion of a one-to-one correspondence between specific linguistic structural elements and focal segments of the brain. Separate levels of description are nec-

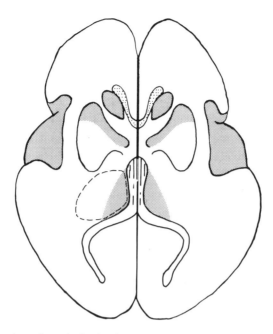

FIG. 2.13. Posterior subcortical aphasia, horizontal view

essary for elements of language and for neurobiological systems, and these separate levels are only loosely coupled.

A comprehensive neurologic theory of language must take into account evidence that most parts of the brain are engaged in the language act. Neuroimaging studies of normal volunteers stand in stark contrast with clinicopathological studies of aphasic patients. For example, in normal subjects observed for simple noise discriminations, cerebral activation is seen in *both* hemispheres, primarily in the temporal lobes. With even the slightest increase in linguistic complexity, whether it be for discrimination, comprehension, or production, cerebral activation extends widely, including both sylvian regions and both prefrontal regions, and especially involving the left posterior inferior frontal region.

With aphasic subjects, neuroimaging studies of static lesions, such as computerized axial tomography, have tended to support the classical views of highly localized correlates of language disorder. In contrast, cerebral activation studies, such as cerebral blood flow studies, document regional cerebral involvement in selected language activities.

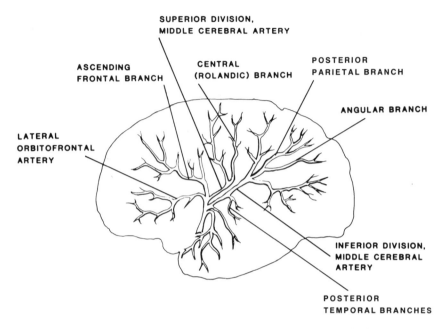

FIG. 2.14. Blood supply to zone of language: branches of middle cerebral artery

Thus, strong evidence now exists to support each of three apparently conflicting views of the neurology of language: (a) that elements of language can be related to highly focal cerebral centers, (b) that language is organized in the brain in a regional or zone-like pattern, and (c) that every language act involves networks of neurons widely distributed throughout the brain, functioning in series and in parallel.

It is possible to accommodate these three notions in a single model, based on one developed by Bachman and Albert (1990). Multiple, complex overlapping neuronal systems most likely are involved in language processing. These neuronal networks include cortical and subcortical components, some of which are near each other, providing the basis for regional contributions to language, and some of which are more distant, providing the basis for widely distributed, parallel processing of aspects of language. All of the regional and widely distributed networks are multiply interconnected.

Within the classical "zone of language," extensive superimposition occurs of the neural networks critical to language. These areas of multiple overlap may correspond to what was called in classical neurology the "centers" of language. Instead of serving as storage centers for language, however, which is the classical notion, they may represent critical "bottlenecks" for the processing of selected elements of language. A focal lesion in one of these critical locations could produce a predictable aphasic deficit.

As will emerge in subsequent chapters, this view of the neurology of language not only enhances understanding the phenomena of recovery from aphasia, but also lends itself readily to the development of theoretically motivated, brain-based approaches to aphasia therapy.

References and Selected Readings

Alexander, M.P., Naeser, M.A., & Palumbo, C.L. (1987). Correlations of subcortical CT lesion sites and aphasia profiles. *Brain, 110,* 961–991.

Bachman, D., & Albert, M.L. (1990). The cerebral organization of language. In A. Peters & E. Jones (Eds.), *Cerebral cortex.* New York: Plenum.

Benson, D.F. (1979). *Aphasia, alexia, agraphia.* New York: Churchill Livingston.

Geschwind, N. (1965). Disconnexion syndromes in animals and man. *Brain, 88,* 237–294, 585–644.

Kertesz, A. (Ed.). (1983). *Localization in neuropsychology.* New York: Academic Press.

Classification
of Aphasia

The aphasia classification systems used most commonly by aphasiologists include the following syndromes, broadly grouped as "cortical" or "subcortical" according to the major site of the responsible brain lesion:

"Cortical" Syndromes
Broca's aphasia
Wernicke's aphasia
Conduction aphasia
Anomic aphasia
Transcortical motor aphasia
Transcortical sensory aphasia
Global aphasia

"Subcortical" Syndromes
Anterior capsular/putaminal aphasia
Posterior capsular/putaminal aphasia
Global capsular/putaminal aphasia
Thalamic aphasia

As many as 80% of patients whose aphasia results from a stroke can be classified according to this system. Some unclassifiable forms of aphasia may be accounted for by such factors as unusual combinations of lesion sites within the left hemisphere, atypical cerebral dominance with left-handedness or ambidexterity, or a positive neurological history, which might include previous strokes, carotid insufficiency, or substance abuse. Because these same factors may influence recovery patterns, this information should be obtained for all patients, even those whose aphasia is easily classifiable.

The aphasia classification system described in this chapter relates primarily to the acquired language disorders resulting from left cerebral stroke. In most cases there will be a history of sudden onset, often with concomitant right-sided weakness or paralysis, following which these symptoms become stable or improve. If instead there is slow onset of speech/language problems with continued deterioration, then an etiology other than stroke (e.g., dementia, brain tumor, vasculitis, encephalitis) should be considered and investigated.

I. Differential Diagnosis of the "Cortical" Aphasia Syndromes

The so-called "cortical" syndromes can be differentially diagnosed on the basis of strengths and weakness in four speech/language skills: naming, conversational speech fluency, auditory comprehension, and word/sentence repetition.

A. Determining the Presence of Naming Problems

All aphasic patients have naming problems; that is, they have difficulty retrieving or producing certain labels. The first step in the differential diagnosis of aphasia, therefore, is to establish the presence of a naming disorder, called **anomia**. Anomia is seldom a pervasive phenomenon. Some aphasia patients, for example, have difficulty in naming low frequency objects, such as *telescope*. Other patients have impaired naming for specific semantic categories, such as body parts and colors. Performance also may be influenced by the nature of the task, so that confrontation naming (i.e., "What is this?") may be easier than free recall (e.g., "Name as many animals as possible"). In establishing the presence of anomia, all of these factors should be addressed (word frequency, semantic category, nature of naming task). The process is summarized as follows:

Patient With Stroke

↓

Battery of Naming Tests

Confrontation naming of objects (high to low frequency)
actions (high to low frequency)
letters
numbers
colors
body parts

Free recall naming of animals

↓

Abnormal Naming Performance

↓

Aphasic Patient

B. Determining Speech Fluency

The next step in the differential diagnosis of aphasia is the determination of speech fluency. The cortical aphasias can be subdivided into two forms, **fluent aphasia** and **nonfluent apha-**

sia, based on characteristics of conversational speech. The conversational sample obtained should include speech elicited in response to social interactions (e.g., "How are you today?") and to personally relevant questions requiring both short and longer answers (e.g., "What do you do for a living?" or "What happened to bring you here?"). This sample should be tape-recorded for careful analysis, although the experienced clinician may make reliable informal judgments "on-line."

There are six conversational speech parameters to be considered. Four of these can be judged objectively from a transcription:

1. **Phrase length:** the number of words uttered in a breath unit.

2. **Substantive/functor word balance:** the normal ratio of both high information (content/substantive) words and functor (grammatical) words versus a prevalence of either substantive or functor words.

3. **Syntax use:** the production of syntactic constructions.

4. **Paraphasia:** the occurrence and prevalence of paraphasias, including:

    a. **Literal/phonemic paraphasias** (e.g., *stoon* for *spoon*)

    b. **Verbal/semantic paraphasias** (e.g., *knife* for *spoon*)

    c. **Neologistic paraphasias** (e.g., *stoffle* for *spoon*)

The two additional speech parameters must be judged subjectively because they are qualitative measures:

5. **Speech prosody:** the intonation or melody of normal speech.

6. **Articulatory agility:** the ease and precision with which the connected sounds of speech are produced without struggle or distortion.

The following overview represents the process of determining speech fluency in an aphasic patient:

Rating a Conversational Speech Sample

1 2 3   4   5 6 7

Phrase Length
Single Words. . . . . 7 or More Words

Substantive/Functor Word Balance
Mostly Substantives. . . . . Mostly Functors

Grammatical Form
None . . . . Normal Range

Paraphasias
Rare . . . . Frequent

Speech Prosody
Severely Impaired . . . . Normal

Articulatory Agility
Severely Impaired . . . . Normal

If the ratings on the majority of these conversational measures fall either at the center (a rating of 4) or to the left of center, the diagnosis is nonfluent aphasia. If most of the ratings are to the right of center, a diagnosis of fluent aphasia is made. In some syndromes, however, one of these parameters may deviate from the fluent/nonfluent feature dichotomy. This is especially true of some of the subcortical syndromes, as will be explained. Patients who produce very little speech or only a stereotypy (e.g., "bika-bika," "fifty-fifty") cannot be rated according to a conversational speech profile. In general, the various aphasias fall into the fluent/nonfluent categories as follows:

Nonfluent Aphasia	*Fluent Aphasia*
Broca's	Wernicke's
Transcortical Motor	Transcortical Sensory
Global	Anomic
	Conduction

C. Determining Auditory Comprehension Skills

Auditory comprehension rarely is entirely preserved in aphasia, but in some nonfluent and fluent aphasia syndromes auditory comprehension is *relatively* better than speech production. In other syndromes, auditory comprehension is no better or worse than speech production. Thus, auditory comprehension can be used to arrive at a more precise diagnosis than the broad classifications of fluent or nonfluent aphasia. A summary of the factors that are addressed in the assessment of auditory comprehension skills follows:

Battery of Auditory Comprehension Tests

Single-word identification of objects (high to low frequency)
actions (high to low frequency)
letters
numbers
colors
body parts

Following commands: single-step, naturalistic actions
two-, three-, four-step, unusual actions

Understanding questions related to personal information
impersonal information
everyday stories
paragraphs of obscure facts

Nonfluent Aphasia   **Fluent Aphasia**

Poor	Good	Poor	Good
Auditory	Auditory	Auditory	Auditory
Comprehen.	Comprehen.	Comprehen.	Comprehen.
↓	↓	↓	↓
Global	Broca's	Wernicke's	Conduction
	Transcortical	Transcortical	Anomic
	Motor	Sensory	

In testing auditory comprehension, it is important to assess the patient's ability to understand spoken single-word commands as well as sentences and paragraph-length material requiring yes/no responses. Furthermore, as in naming, comprehension at the single-word level may be influenced by such factors as word finding and semantic class. For example, some patients show relatively better comprehension for action words versus object names. Among the factors to consider in giving commands is that comprehension for naturalistic, single-step commands (e.g., "Close your eyes" or "Stand up") may be good, while comprehension for unusual, multistep comments (e.g., "Put the pen on top of the card" or "Tap your left shoulder once using two fingers") may be partially or totally impaired. Similarly, comprehension of personally relevant questions (e.g., "Is your name _____?"") may be good, while comprehension of nonpersonal questions (e.g., "Is the sky blue?") may be impaired. Short paragraphs that relate everyday events (e.g., a flat tire on a vacation trip) are easier to understand than longer paragraphs of unfamiliar, formal information (e.g., the nest-building practices of snowy egrets). All of these factors should be addressed in the assessment of auditory comprehension skills.

D. Determining Repetition Skills

Global aphasia is differentially diagnosed as the probable syndrome in a patient with little or no speech output and poor auditory comprehension; the task of *repetition* is used to differentiate the remaining six cortical aphasia syndromes. As with auditory comprehension, it is important to consider the *relative* preservation or disturbance of repetition skills, vis-à-vis conversational speech ability. Fluent and nonfluent patients may show patterns of relatively good or poor repetition skills when this ability is weighed against their ability to produce similar speech units in conversation.

Tests of repetition skill should include single words, phrases, and sentences. Single words should represent a variety of semantic categories of both high and low frequency words. In addition to the semantic categories used in naming and auditory comprehension, the list should include functor words such as *if.* Word repetition tests also should include single-syllable, phonetically simple words, such as *babe,* as well as multisyllable, phonetically more complex words, such as *kitchen.* The emotional value of a word may influence performance, so that words such as *love* may be easy to repeat. Phrase and sentence repetition should begin with short, everyday phrases (e.g., "Sit down") and progress to longer utterances, such as "He has decided to stay overnight." These can be compared with infrequently occurring, short (e.g., "Lobsters molt") and long (e.g., "Thermodynamics deals with the mechanical actions of heat") sentences.

The following diagram summarizes this diagnostic process:

Battery of Repetition Tests

Single words, representing a variety of semantic categories
high and low frequency
emotional and neutral valence
single and multisyllables
phonetic variation

Phrases and sentences, representing short everyday phrases
longer everyday sentences
short unfamiliar phrases
long unfamiliar phrases

Nonfluent Aphasia   Fluent Aphasia

Good Auditory Comprehension	Poor Auditory Comprehension	Good Auditory Comprehension
Poor Repetition — Good Repetition	Poor Repetition — Good Repetition	Poor Repetition — Good Repetition
Broca's — Transcortical Motor	Wernicke's — Transcortical Sensory	Conduction — Anomic

An overview of the complete cortical aphasia diagnostic "tree" is presented in Fig. 3.1.

II. Differential Diagnosis of the "Subcortical" Aphasias

As shown, the seven cortical aphasia syndromes can be differentially diagnosed on the basis of four speech/language behaviors: naming, conversational speech fluency, auditory comprehension, and repetition. In diagnosing the "subcortical" syndromes, three additional behaviors are considered:

1. **Verbal agility:** the ability to repeat words or short phrases rapidly (e.g., "papa, papa, papa, etc." or "pink panther, pink panther, etc.") up to 10 times in 1 minute. Poor performance may result either from poor articulatory agility (effortful, imprecise articulation) or from intrusion of phonemic or neologistic paraphasias.

2. **Nonverbal agility:** the ability to produce precise nonvocal, oral movements rapidly (e.g., protruding-retracting the tongue).

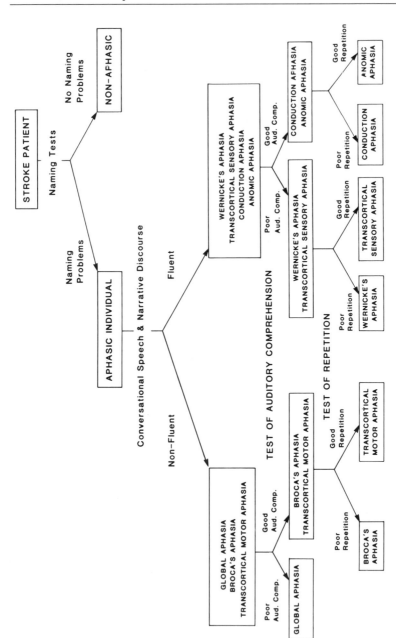

FIG. 3.1. Classification of "cortical" aphasia syndromes

3. **Hemiplegia/hemiparesis:** paralysis/weakness of the right side of the body in right-handers.

To understand the features of the subcortical syndromes, it is necessary first to consider the neuropathology of these syndromes vis-à-vis the pathways between subcortical structures and the cortical areas associated with the seven cortical aphasia syndromes (these pathways are described in chapters 1 and 2).

A. Anterior Capsular/Putaminal Aphasia

A lesion in the anterior portion of the internal capsule will interrupt speech production and speech initiation pathways from the areas associated with Broca's and transcortical motor aphasia (see chapter 2). Such a lesion will produce a syndrome that has features of both transcortical motor and Broca's aphasia. The features of anterior capsular/putaminal aphasia are outlined in Fig. 3.2.

B. Posterior Capsular/Putaminal Aphasia

A lesion in the posterior portion of the internal capsule will interrupt auditory pathways to the cortical area associated with Wernicke's aphasia as well as motor pathways from the motor cortex. Such a lesion will produce a syndrome that has features of both Broca's and Wernicke's aphasia. The features of posterior capsular/putaminal aphasia also are outlined in Fig. 3.2.

C. Global Capsular/Putaminal Aphasia

Whereas the cortical global aphasia syndrome requires an extensive lesion involving all of the primary language areas (see chapter 2), a global-like syndrome can result from a relatively small, anterior and posterior capsular/putaminal lesion. Such a subcortical lesion will interrupt pathways to cortical speech comprehension areas and from speech production areas, so that the patient has poor auditory comprehension and little or no verbal output.

D. Thalamic Aphasia

As described in chapter 1, thalamic pathways project to and from both frontal and posterior portions of the cortical language zone and to the motor cortex. A lesion in the thalamus, therefore, may result in a syndrome that has features of both

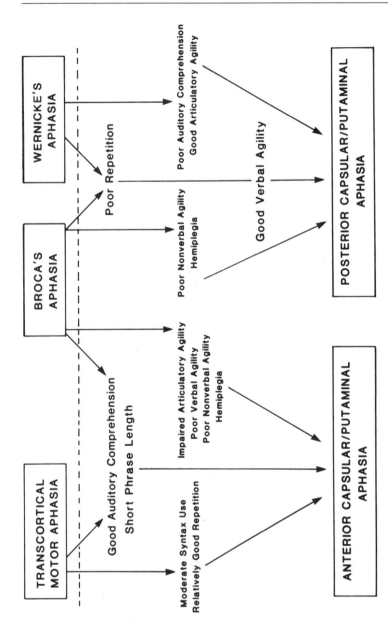

FIG. 3.2. Classification of capsular/putaminal syndromes vis-à-vis "cortical" aphasia syndromes

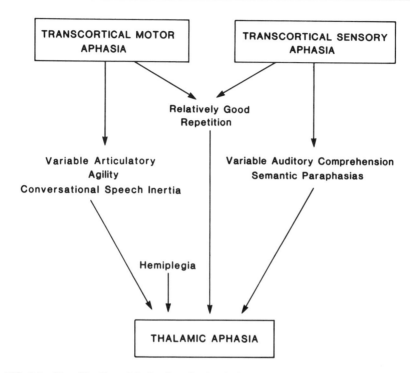

FIG. 3.3. Classification of thalamic aphasia vis-à-vis transcortical syndromes

transcortical motor and transcortical sensory aphasia with hemiplegia. The features of thalamic aphasia are outlined in Fig. 3.3.

In addition to the features outlined in Figs. 3.2 and 3.3, two additional behaviors are seen commonly in the subcortical aphasias and rarely in the cortical syndromes: **hypophonia** and **variable performance**.

III. Unclassifiable Patients

As indicated, perhaps as many as 80% of aphasic patients can be classified as having most or all of the features common to one of the cortical or subcortical aphasia syndromes. Unclassifiable patterns may be accounted for by one or more of the following:

1. **Atypical cerebral dominance**, as suggested by a personal or family history of left-handedness or ambidexterity or learning disability, or by "reversed" occipital lobe asym-

metries (i.e., longer and wider right than left occipital lobe as measured on CT scan).

2. **Bilateral brain damage**, as suggested by such signs as dysphagia (swallowing problems), persistent incontinence, right- and left-sided weakness, pseudobulbar affect (uncontrolled crying or laughing), severely impaired visual/spatial skills, and/or denial of illness.

3. **Different lesion site combinations** within the dominant left hemisphere.

4. **Progressive neurological disease**, as suggested by deteriorating performance.

5. **Substance abuse**, as suggested by a history of prolonged use of alcohol and/or prescribed and nonprescribed drugs.

When patients do display profiles of speech-language characteristics that allow them to be easily classified, then a diagnostic label such as "Broca's aphasia" is a good reference point for all those working with that individual. For treatment purposes, however, it probably is more important to identify individual strengths and weaknesses than to assign a diagnostic label. This approach will be elaborated upon in subsequent chapters.

Selected Readings

Albert, M.L., Goodglass, H., Helm, N.A., Rubens, A., & Alexander, M.P. (1981). *Clinical aspects of dysphasia.* New York: Springer.

Goodglass, H., & Kaplan, E. (1984). *Assessment of aphasia and related disorders.* Philadelphia: Lea & Febiger.

Section Two
Diagnostic Process

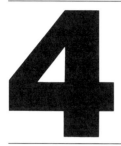

Neurologic
Examination

Accurate diagnosis and competent treatment of aphasia demand an understanding of the patient's medical, neurological, and psychological status. At the very least, a clinician should be sensitive to the possibility that factors other than aphasia may be interfering with recovery of function. Although this statement may seem obvious, clinical experience shows that some aphasic patients considered to be treatment failures ultimately have regained useful language skills after their previously unrecognized epilepsy or digitalis intoxication or reactive depression, or other medical problem, was recognized and properly treated. A review of the neurologic examination and relevant segments of the general medical examination follows.

I. Neurologic History

Even in an era of sophisticated neuroimaging technology, a well-taken history is critical to accurate diagnosis. Three examples, chosen arbitrarily from everyday practice, readily illustrate this point.

1. Some aphasia-producing disorders, such as migraine or epilepsy, may not be associated with identifiable physical findings. The prodrome of a migraine attack, for example, may include an aphasia syndrome, yet no evidence of the underlying abnormality would be found on CT or MRI scans. Similarly, varying patterns of aphasia may be the consequence of a focal epileptic episode. The diagnosis in these cases would be made by history.

2. Some drugs used to treat hypertension may cause depression, which can influence language function. A carefully obtained medical history may provide the first clues to the correct diagnosis.

3. A progressive dementing disorder with difficulties in communication may be associated with the AIDS virus, which in turn may be suspected if a careful social history is obtained.

The following list outlines cardinal features of a neurologic history:

1. **Chief complaint:** statement of problem.

2. **History of present illness:** logical, sequential reconstruction of onset and progression of symptoms.

3. **Review of neurologic complaints:** detailed evaluation of symptoms referable to each major component of central and peripheral nervous systems (e.g., headache, dizziness, pain, weakness, syncope, etc.).

4. **Review of systems:** detailed evaluation of symptoms referable to each major organ system (cardiovascular, renal, etc.).

5. **Medical history:** review of major illnesses (e.g., diabetes, hypertension, cardiovascular illness, endocrine abnormalities, psychiatric disability, head injury, congenital abnormality, significant childhood illness, etc.); special emphasis on developmental learning disorders; use of any medications.

6. **Family history:** pertinent medical, neurological, or psychiatric illnesses, as well as handedness (in patient and family).

7. **Social history:** educational and social development; occupations (for possibility of toxic exposure); nutritional habits and status (for possibility of deficiency syndromes); alcohol and drug use.

II. Neurologic Examination

Observation is the clinical basis of a good neurologic examination. Key elements of the neurologic examination can be carried out indirectly, by astute observation of how the patient walks into the room, shakes hands, sits, presents the history, etc. It is not an exaggeration, for example, to state that a major portion of the mental status examination can be completed while the neurologic history is being taken.

The neurologic examination is a systematic clinical analysis of the major components of the central and peripheral nervous systems, outlined as follows: (a) general observations and medical examination, (b) mental status examination, (c) cranial nerves, (d) motor system, (e) reflexes, and (f) sensation.

A. General Observations and Medical Examination

Some items described here under "general observations" might just as easily be included under "mental status examination" or "motor system." However, the preference implied here is to conduct as much of the neurologic examination as one can indirectly. General observations include the following:

1. **Behavior:** level and type of social interaction, cleanliness, neatness, dress, affect, mood, thought processes, anxiety, confusion, sense of humor, type of humor, appropriateness, delusions, hallucinations.

2. **Gait and posture:** evidence of asymmetry, weakness, unsteadiness, abnormalities of gait (e.g., circumduction of one leg may indicate hemiparesis; festination may indicate Parkinson's disease; ataxia may indicate cerebellar disease or abnormality in the posterior portions of the spinal cord).

3. **Skin, head, neck, and spine:** moles, lumps, rashes, or discolorations of the skin (may point to specific neurologic diseases, such as congenital abnormalities of the brain, neurofibromatosis, etc.); large, low-set ears, excessively wide or narrow distance between the eyes, or other abnormalities of the head or face (may signal underlying cerebral abnormalities); asymmetries of pulsation or bruits in carotid arteries, as revealed by gentle palpation and listening through a stethoscope (may suggest vascular disease); spinal scoliosis or moles or dimples at base of spine (may reflect associated neurologic disease, such as abnormalities of spinal cord development).

The "medical examination" should include detailed testing of any medical system for which complaints were elicited during history taking. In addition, examine blood pressure in both arms with the patient recumbent and standing.

B. Mental Status Examination

There are probably as many approaches to the mental status examination as examiners. However, two standards of evaluation in particular are useful: (a) in testing each component of mental status, try to be as supportive and encouraging as possible; and (b) while being constantly concerned for the psychological well-being of the patient, try to be rather strict. In applying both standards to an individual patient, one may be able to gauge the limits of the patient's capabilities; that is, the best and worst performances for each cognitive skill.

A bedside mental status examination includes the following elements (more detailed descriptions of language and neuropsychological examinations are provided in subsequent chapters):

1. **General level of mental function:** awake, alert, attentive, appropriate.

2. **Memory:** immediate recall (e.g., digit span), recent memory (e.g., awareness of current events, ability to learn four unrelated items and recall them after 5 minutes), remote memory (e.g., awareness of major events in past history).

3. **Language:** spontaneous speech, naming, comprehension, repetition, reading, writing.

4. **Visuospatial functions:** drawing to copy and command; spatial orientation (e.g., how does the patient get around in his or her environment?).

5. **Manipulation of acquired knowledge:** problem solving, proverb interpretation, complex calculations.

C. Cranial Nerves

There are 12 cranial nerves:

1. Olfactory
2. Optic
3. Oculomotor
4. Trochlear
5. Trigeminal
6. Abducens
7. Facial
8. Acoustic
9. Glossopharyngeal
10. Vagus
11. Spinal accessory
12. Hypoglossal

Students often develop mnemonics to facilitate recollection of these nerves. A popular such device is "On Old Olympus's Towering Tops, A Fair Armed Goddess Viewed Some Hops." Table 4.1 provides a brief review of functions and tests for the cranial nerves.

D. Motor System

In addition to gait and posture (discussed under section II.A. "General Observations"), one should test tone, bulk, strength, and coordination, and observe the patient for signs of involuntary movements. In all testing, look especially for asymmetries.

1. **Tone:** Look for evidence of increased or decreased tone by passively flexing and extending limbs at major joints. **Spasticity** (often a long-term consequence of a cerebral hemispheric stroke) is increased tone in antigravity muscles; **rigidity** is increased tone in both **agonists** (muscles that are the prime movers; i.e., they act to produce the desired movement) and **antagonists** (muscles that act to counter the agonists). For a movement to be smooth, when agonists contract, antagonists relax. Look also for intermittent, ratchet-like rigidity (i.e., "cogwheeling," a common feature of Parkinson's disease).

2. **Bulk:** Look for signs of selective or generalized muscle wasting or hypertrophy (such abnormalities may reflect primary muscle disease).

3. **Strength:** Look expecially for signs of selective or asymmetric weakness. Usually, neurologic diseases do not cause generalized weakness; rather, they are more likely to cause specific patterns of muscle weakness (e.g., hemiplegia, shoulder girdle weakness, etc.). Complaints of generalized weakness usually derive from non-neurological illnesses (e.g., influenza, anemia, depression). Test muscle groups across all major joints, in flexion, extension, abduction, and adduction. In reporting results, the names of specific muscles are not necessary; it is sufficient just to indicate the affected muscle group and the degree of weakness. For example, one might develop a scale for degree of weakness, with "0" representing no strength and "5" representing full strength. Thus, if strength is moderately impaired in the right shoulder, one would report "strength reduced to 3 out of 5 at right shoulder."

TABLE 4.1
Cranial Nerves

Cranial nerve	Function	Test
Olfactory	Sense of smell	Occlude one nostril and ask patient to close eyes. Test each nostril separately with common aromatic substances, such as coffee. Avoid irritants, such as ammonia.
Optic	Vision	Test visual acuity and visual fields. Optic fundi should be examined for signs of abnormality.
Oculomotor Trochlear Abducens	Function together as an integrated system for eye movements, eyelid elevation, and constriction of pupils	Eyes are "yoked," so they should move in a balanced, symmetrical manner. Ask patient to move eyes in all directions (voluntary control) and to follow fingers in all directions (tracking). Look for drooping of eyelids and response of pupils to light.
Trigeminal	Control of chewing, sensation on face, and corneal reflex	Ask patient to open and close jaw. Test for weakness or deviation of jaw. Test facial sensation; look for asymmetries. Touch outer edge of cornea with cotton wisp.
Facial	Control of muscles of facial expression	Test voluntary (i.e., response to examiner request) and automatic (i.e., response to natural conversation, joke, etc.) control of expression (e.g., smile, frown, and eye closure).
Acoustic	Hearing, balance, and equilibrium	Test hearing in each ear by rubbing fingers near ears. Compare with audition for ticking of a watch. Look at eyes for nystagmus at rest, on lateral or up/down gaze, and after shaking head.
Glossopharyngeal	Sensation to pharynx and posterior one third of tongue	Touch back of oral cavity with tongue depressor or cotton swab. Look for hyperactive or hypoactive gag reflex or asymmetry of reflex.
Vagus	Motor control of palate, pharynx, and larynx	Look at palate for drooping or asymmetry. When patient says "aahh," look for deviation of uvula. Listen for hoarseness (ask if it is of recent onset). Otherwise, test as for glossopharyngeal nerve.
Spinal accessory	Head turning and shoulder shrugging	Place your hand against patient's chin and cheek. Ask patient to turn his/her head against the resistance of your hand. (Head turning to right is a test of the left sternocleidomastoid muscle, and vice versa.) Ask patient to shrug shoulders against the resistance of your hands.
Hypoglossal	Control of tongue movement	Look at tongue for abnormal movements or signs of wasting. Ask patient to stick out tongue in midline (look for deviation from midline) and to move it from side to side. A good test is to ask patient to "lick your lips all around."

4. **Coordination:** Cerebellar dysfunction can produce impairments of coordination. Do not confuse weakness with impaired coordination. Observe the patient's balance when walking and sitting. Have the patient touch your finger and then touch his or her nose several times in succession with each hand. Look for clumsy or misdirected movements. Have the patient run the heel (shoes off) of one foot up and down the shin of the other leg. Look for awkwardness and shakiness.

5. **Involuntary movements:** Look for any evidence of involuntary shaking, twitching, tremor, or twisting of any part of the body.

E. Reflexes

Test **deep tendon reflexes** (i.e., muscle stretch reflexes) and **pathological** or **release reflexes**. To test deep tendon reflexes, strike the tendons with a reflex hammer, thereby rapidly stretching the associated muscle. For purposes of the aphasia-related examination, it is sufficient to test the biceps reflex, the wrist reflex, the knee jerk, and the ankle jerk. Look for asymmetry, hyperactivity, or hypoactivity. Damage to upper (cortical) motor neurons often will produce contralateral hyperactivity of reflexes. Damage to lower motor neurons (in the spinal cord) will reduce muscle stretch reflexes, causing hypoactivity.

So-called pathological reflexes are normal in infants and usually disappear in the first or second year of life. Some of them may reappear with normal aging. In the years from childhood through middle age, their presence usually denotes evidence of dysfunction in the central nervous system.

1. **The Babinski sign** indicates dysfunction in the pyramidal tract. Stroke the lateral aspect of the sole of the foot, starting at the heel, and running the stimulus across the ball of the foot. Stimulation should be slow, steady, and mildly noxious. A key is a useful device for this purpose. A normal response is flexion of the toes. A pathological response is extension of the large toe with spreading of the other toes, hence the frequently used term "up-going toes."

2. **Snout reflex:** Tap the upper lip. A puckering response is abnormal.

3. **Rooting reflex:** Tap the cheek. An involuntary movement of the angle of the mouth toward the tap is abnormal. These signs suggest frontal lobe dysfunction.

4. **Grasp reflex:** Gently stroke the web between the thumb and first finger of the patient's relaxed hand. An abnormal response is an involuntary grasp of the stroking fingers. This response usually indicates contralateral frontal lobe disease.

F. Sensation

The traditional approach to sensory testing, also used here, divides sensation roughly into two categories: **primary** and **cortical**. This approach is highly schematic and necessarily incomplete. The primary sensory modalities include touch, pain, temperature, vibration, and position. Included within the cortical sensations are two-point discrimination, stereognosis, and graphesthesia. (In fact, cortical, spinal cord, and peripheral nerve mechanisms are all involved in reception and interpretation of external stimuli. It would be inappropriate, for example, to attempt to evaluate impaired two-point discrimination without first taking into account sensation for light touch and pain.)

Table 4.2 briefly summarizes the sensory examination. As always in neurology, look especially for asymmetries, not only left/right, but also proximal/distal and upper body/lower body. The nervous system provides overlapping sensory areas. Thus, it would be most unusual for a sensory deficit to have a sharp border.

Psychological factors such as anxiety, depression, or even just fatigue can influence a patient's response and must always be taken into account. As the nervous system provides overlapping sensory areas, graded or blurry edges, rather than sharp edges, should be expected for regions of decreased sensation. It would be most unusual, on a strictly neurologic basis, for someone to have a hemi-anesthesia that comes directly to the midline ("splits the midline") and stops abruptly. Fading of sensation 1 or 2 inches across the midline is more likely. "Splitting the midline" would make the examiner think of possible psychogenic sensory loss (e.g., conversion reaction).

In most cases in neurology, a carefully taken history and physical examination will lead to the correct clinical diagnosis.

TABLE 4.2
Sensory Examination

Modalities	Test	Neuroanatomic region tested
PRIMARY		
Light touch	Cotton swab or light finger pressure on symmetrical regions of body	Both posterior columns and spinothalamic tracts
Pain	Pinprick (jab *very* gently; do not draw blood; always use new, sterile needle)	Spinothalamic tracts
Temperature	Contrast any cold object (e.g., side of tuning fork) with any warmer object (e.g., tongue depressor or pencil)	Spinothalamic tracts
Vibration	Tuning fork, preferably 128 Hz, on bony prominences	Posterior columns
Position (joint position sense)	Hold individual phalanges (fingers, toes) gently on each side and move up or down slowly. Ask when the movement begins.	Posterior columns
CORTICAL		
Two-point discrimination	Simultaneously touch regions of skin with two pins close together but not touching. (See cautionary remarks above on testing for pain.) Repeat test with pins slightly more separated. Repeat test until patient identifies two distinct pins. Note distance between pins. Compare with homologous region on other side of body.	*
Stereognosis	Ask patient to close his/her eyes and identify objects placed in hand. Patient may manipulate object or examiner may move object across the hand.	*
Graphesthesia	Using his/her own index finger, examiner writes numbers on different parts of patient's body—palm, back, etc. With eyes closed, patient must identify numbers.	*

*All cortical somesthetic modalities are presumed to be mediated by parietal association cortex.

Additional diagnostic tests that will aid in determining the nature and extent of neurologic dysfunction are discussed in the next chapter.

Selected Readings

DeJong, R. (1979). *The neurologic examination* (4th ed.). New York: Harper & Row.

Denny-Brown, D. (1982). *Handbook of neurologic examination and case recording* (3rd ed.). Cambridge, MA: Harvard University Press.

Strub, R., & Black, F. (1977). *The mental status examination in neurology*. Philadelphia: F.A. Davis.

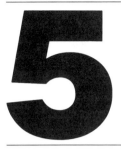

Neurodiagnostic Techniques

Several common diagnostic tests can help define the location of a cerebral lesion, the nature or pathological characteristics of the lesion, and the regions of the brain that have not been damaged. Today most patients hospitalized for suspicion of a cerebral lesion will receive a CT scan (computerized axial tomography) of the brain, an EEG (electroencephalogram), and an LP (lumbar puncture) with examination of the CSF (cerebrospinal fluid). Additional diagnostic techniques, such as magnetic resonance imaging or cerebral angiography, may be used if appropriate to the medical condition and if available in the hospital.

I. Standard Neurodiagnostic Procedures

A. Cerebrospinal Fluid Examination

Cerebrospinal fluid (CSF) fills the ventricles and washes through the subarachnoid space, bathing and protecting the brain. Damage to brain tissue from tumor, infection, stroke, and so forth may be reflected in changes in the composition of CSF. A lumbar puncture (LP) may be done to remove a small amount of CSF for laboratory analysis. Ordinarily one would not carry out a lumbar puncture if there were suspicion of increased intracranial pressure, due, for example, to the presence of a space-occupying lesion in the brain. An LP in such a case might result in herniation of the brain, that is, a sudden forceful downward pressure of the brain through narrow openings in the skull, causing compression of brain tissue. When a space-occupying lesion is suspected, a CT scan ordinarily is taken first, before an LP is done.

To carry out a lumbar puncture, a long, small-bore needle is inserted into the lumbar subarachnoid space. A pressure measuring device attached to the needle can be used to measure the intracranial pressure. Small amounts of CSF, generally 5–10 ml, are removed and analyzed for the presence and amount of cells, sugar, protein, and other elements.

Lumbar puncture is particularly useful if infection of the brain is suspected. Subarachnoid hemorrhage, tumor, and multiple sclerosis are among the many other neurological conditions for which CSF analysis may be helpful.

B. Electroencephalography

Neuronal activity is bioelectric, and this electrical activity of the brain can be measured with electroencephalography (EEG). Electrodes are attached to the patient's scalp, in a placement pattern agreed to by international convention. The electrodes are attached at the other end to a machine that amplifies and records the rhythmic electrical activity of the brain (brain waves).

Rhythmic electrical patterns of brain activity vary in different regions of the brain. In posterior regions (occipital, parietal, posterior temporal) there is ordinarily a symmetrical brain wave frequency of 8–12 cycles per second, called **alpha waves**. In the frontal region one often sees a symmetric, slightly faster, lower amplitude brain wave activity of 14–20 cycles per second, called **beta waves**. As the patient becomes drowsy, a slower wave pattern of 4–6 cycles per second, called **theta waves**, emerges typically in the anterior to mid-temporal regions. Additional wave forms appear in various stages of sleep and in other conditions of normal function, such as sudden arousal.

Asymmetries of wave forms between the two hemispheres, abnormal or unexpected slowing of wave forms, and sharp, rapid, high-voltage wave forms (called **spike discharges** or **spikes**) are among the findings sought by the electroencephalographer in defining brain disease. A patient with epilepsy, for example, may have an abundance of spike discharges from a small subset of electrodes, implying the presence of an epileptic focus in the brain under those electrodes. A patient with structural damage to brain cells, as can occur with a stroke or brain tumor, may have an asymmetrical pattern of high-voltage, very slow waves of 2–4 cycles per second (called **delta waves**), with the slow activity occurring just above the damaged brain tissue. Symmetrical slow wave activity in the theta-delta range occurring bifrontally may be a sign of metabolic encephalopathy.

Artefacts and normal electrical changes must not be confused with abnormal brain waves. Eye movements, respiration, other muscle activity, heart beat, and so forth all may cause artefacts on the EEG. Normal aging may cause slowing of the usual posterior alpha activity by as much as 1 cycle per second for each decade over age 60.

Because of possible technical and artefactual problems that may creep in, no ancillary diagnostic test should ever be substituted for a careful, thoughtful history and physical examination in arriving at a neurologic diagnosis. Neurodiagnostic technology should be used as an extension of the clinician's personal evaluation of a problem, not as a substitute.

C. Computerized Axial Tomography

Although the field of neuroimaging is in rapid flux, computerized axial tomography (CT scan) of the brain represents the most important technology currently available for localization of cerebral lesions. By means of sophisticated, computer-assisted X-ray technology, a series of X rays of the brain at multiple angles is obtained. X-ray profiles are rapidly added together by the computer, producing cross-sectional images of the brain from various angles with excellent definition of intracerebral structures.

Pathological processes such as stroke or tumor can produce abnormal patterns of radiodensity or may displace normal intracranial structures. Due to recent improvements in technology, precise details of lesion localization can be determined within a few millimeters. Nevertheless, as with all ancillary diagnostic techniques, CT scanning has its limitations. Thrombotic or embolic infarctions may not be seen within the first few days of onset. CT lesion size may evolve over time, getting larger or smaller, due in part to local neuronal factors such as cerebral edema. Very tiny lesions may be missed.

Despite these cautionary notes, CT scanning has contributed considerably to our understanding of aphasia. In general, CT scans have confirmed traditional clinicopathological correlations. In addition, however, CT scanning has helped clarify the nature of atypical aphasias, has created the new diagnostic category of subcortical aphasia, and is helping us explore mechanisms of recovery of function in aphasia.

II. Additional Neurodiagnostic Procedures

Beyond computerized axial tomography, electroencephalography, and cerebrospinal fluid analysis, there are additional, less frequently used neurodiagnostic tests: some that are needed only for highly selected problems, such as cerebral angiography, some that are expensive and not yet available at many hospitals, such as magnetic resonance imaging, and some that are still considered primarily research tools, such as positron emission tomography or regional cerebral blood flow studies. In addition, there is another group of neurodiagnostic techniques which will not be discussed here, either because they have been superseded by alternatives and are no longer popular (e.g., pneumoencephalography; radioisotope brain scanning) or because they are so new that their clinical relevance has not yet been demonstrated (e.g., magnetoencephalography).

A. Magnetic Resonance Imaging

Nuclear magnetic resonance (NMR), as a technique useful for chemical analysis, has been available in biochemistry laboratories since the mid-1940s. Only since the early 1970s, however, has this technique, now called magnetic resonance imaging (MRI), been used as a clinical tool. Because no metal can be put through the MRI scanner, the doctor will ask the patient a few questions about his or her history (e.g., "Do you have any metal plates in your head or any shrapnel in your body? Have you ever worked in a factory with metal fragments?"). The patient is then brought through a metal detector into the scanning room. The patient lies down on a table and the technician helps place the patient's head comfortably into a padded cradle. A clear plastic screen is placed over the patient's head about 10 inches from the face. The patient will hear a noise around his or her head that is very similar to the sound of a washing machine. This procedure continues for approximately 1 to 2 hours.

Magnetic resonance imaging and computerized axial tomography both provide images of the body (hence the label "imaging techniques"); however, the physics and machinery of each are different. CT is an X-ray technique in which many X rays are taken of a body part from different angles, and cross-sectional X-ray shadow images of that body part are represented by means of a computerized reconstruction algorithm. By contrast, MRI uses a strong magnetic field to produce a temporary realignment of the nuclei of atoms in the cells of the tissue being studied (like iron filings lining up and pointing in the same direction when placed near a magnet). Measurements are made of rates of alignment and disalignment of these atomic nuclei when they are subjected to varying amounts of electromagnetic radiation. These rates of nuclear movement are entered into a computer program, which then can construct an image of the relevant tissue.

MRI is superior to CT in certain situations and less useful in others. For example, with ischemic infarction MRI can detect and localize the lesion within a few hours of vascular occlusion, whereas CT evidence may not occur in the first few days. On the other hand, acute cerebral hemorrhage is more reliably demonstrated with CT than with MRI within the first 48 hours. MRI is free from certain artefacts of CT and provides better gray-white matter discrimination and better lesion delineation. However, the value of MRI over CT in the diagnosis and treatment of aphasia remains to be proven.

B. Cerebral Angiography

Although cerebral angiography was once used commonly to help localize and define intracranial mass lesions, this diagnostic technique is being limited more and more to exploration of the blood vessels supplying the brain. The current goals of cerebral angiography include the identification of vascular stenosis or occlusion, cerebral aneurysms or other vascular malformations, and vasculitis.

Typically the process entails inserting a flexible plastic catheter into a femoral artery in the groin and threading it upward through the aortic arch, under fluoroscopic control. In this manner it is possible to place the catheter selectively into the carotid or vertebral arteries. Radio-opaque contrast material is then injected into the chosen blood vessel, and a series of X-ray films is taken rapidly as the dye moves through the arterial system, capillary network, and venous system, thus allowing X-ray visualization of the brain's entire vascular supply.

As with all neurodiagnostic techniques, angiography is not without its risks. Threading the catheter through the blood vessels may dislodge atherosclerotic plaques and cause emboli; a patient may be allergic to the dye; and so forth. This technique may be most dangerous for the people who need it most, those with atherosclerotic or inflammatory disease of cerebral blood vessels. The ratio of possible risk to possible benefit must be weighed carefully in these patients.

C. Positron Emission Tomography

Positron emission tomography (PET) uses CT technology to enable clinicians to visualize cerebral metabolic activity. Microscopic quantities of radioactive chemicals are injected into the patient and patterns of subsequent radioactivity are recorded over the brain. This technique allows in vivo assessment of normal as well as damaged brains, and it has been employed successfully in the study of aphasia. The radioactive chemical is acted on in different cerebral regions in direct proportion to the metabolic demands made on that particular cerebral area. The combination of static anatomical imaging (CT, MRI) and dynamic metabolic imaging (PET) provides extraordinary opportunities for testing neurolinguistic theories.

PET scanning is, nonetheless, subject to technical limitations, such as the relatively poor power of resolution of PET machines, the blurring and distortion of lesion boundaries in ischemic infarctions, and the sensitivity of cerebral metabolic activity to subtle changes in internal or external environment. Presumably these problems will be worked out in time. For the present, however, PET scanning is still used more as a research than a clinical tool.

D. Regional Cerebral Blood Flow

In normal cerebral function, cerebral blood flow (CBF) is regulated by neuronal metabolism. It follows, then, that regional measurements of cerebral blood flow (rCBF) can provide indirect measures of neuronal metabolism in brain regions in which blood flow is determined. In the usual technique, a radioactive tracer substance is administered by inhalation through a mask. The patient's head is surrounded by an array of radioactivity detectors. Regional cerebral metabolic activity thus can be inferred and mapped.

In the past 20 years many rCBF studies have been carried out correlating language activity with cerebral metabolic activity. These studies generally have confirmed the traditional models of aphasia. At the same time they have opened up the possibility that many parts of the brain may be activated during a language act, in addition to the "zone of language" in the left hemisphere. Cerebral blood flow studies also have been used in recovery of function studies, and have provided evidence that the right hemisphere can be involved in some cases of recovery from aphasia.

Selected Readings

Oldendorf, W. (1980). *The quest for an image of the brain.* New York: Raven.

Weisberg, L., Strub, R., & Garcia, C. (1989). *Essentials of clinical neurology* (2nd ed.). Rockville, MD: Aspen.

Influence of Medical and Neurological Illness on Aphasia

The clinician caring for a person with aphasia should be cognizant of ways in which signs and symptoms of aphasia can be affected by the interaction of brain pathology and medical illness or neurological disease. To discuss fully the influence of medical and neurological illness on aphasia would require a textbook-length consideration, as so many medical disorders can affect the patterns and progress of aphasia. The intent here, however, is not to be comprehensive, but practical. Certain common neuropathologic changes or medical conditions, such as stroke, seizure, and brain tumor, can cause or modify the picture of aphasia and will be described in the sections that follow.

I. Cerebrovascular Disease

Although there has been no systematic, national, comprehensive, epidemiologic study of aphasia and its causes, it is estimated that cerebrovascular disease may cause as many as half of all aphasia cases. (Head injury may induce about one third, and tumors, dementing illnesses, and central nervous system infections are among the other causes.) As stroke incidence is declining in the United States due to better control of hypertension and healthier life-styles, head injury is increasing as a cause of aphasia. Approximately 20% of persons with stroke become aphasic. Because about 400,000 new attacks of stroke occur in the United States each year, there are nearly 80,000 new cases of aphasia each year in the United States from stroke alone.

A **stroke** is the sudden onset of a neurological deficit due to abrupt interruption of flow in blood vessels to the brain, caused generally by occlusion or rupture of the blood vessel. Rupture of a blood vessel produces hemorrhage or bleeding into or around the brain. Common causes are hypertension, rupture of an aneurysm or vascular malformation, or certain medical conditions such as leukemia or a regimen of anticoagulant medication.

Occlusion of a blood vessel produces **ischemia** (reduction of oxygen), which may be temporary, as in a **transient ischemic attack (TIA)**. A transient ischemic attack is an acute neurologic deficit of vascular cause lasting, by definition, less than 24 hours. Ischemia also may cause a permanent deficit due to **infarction** (destruction) of brain tissue. **Ischemic infarction** usually results from occlusion of a blood vessel due either to **thrombosis** (progressive narrowing and ultimate occlusion of a localized region of a blood vessel, due most commonly to atherosclerosis) or to **embolus** (a blood clot broken off from a blood vessel in one part of the arterial system that travels to another, narrower part of the arterial system and lodges there either temporarily or permanently). Other causes of occlusion are **vasculitis** (inflammation of blood vessels) or invasion of a blood vessel by **tumor**.

Different aphasia syndromes result not only from selective involvement of different blood vessels, as discussed in chapter 1, but also from different etiologies of vascular disease. Different rates and patterns of recovery may be expected as well. For example, **hypertensive intracerebral hemorrhage** usually originates in subcortical gray matter (thalamus or putamen). These strokes may be violent, massive, and serious, often rupturing into the ventricular system and affecting consciousness. If the patient survives, he or she is usually left with a dense hemiplegia and, if the dominant hemisphere is involved, a subcortical aphasia. Recovery from subcortical aphasia, however, regardless of how severe the language loss at first, may be surprisingly good.

One of the factors that may impede recovery from aphasia is the presence of additional brain damage in the nondominant hemisphere. Frequently, persons with hypertension will develop **lacunar infarctions**. These are small (less than 2 cm) areas of infarction resulting from occlusion of small arteries due to changes in the walls of these arteries caused by high blood pressure. The **lacunes**, as they are called, are often bilateral and are located deep in frontal lobe periventricular white matter or in the subcortical gray matter (basal ganglia or thalamus).

A **lacunar state** results from the accumulation of multiple small subcortical lacunar infarctions. In its severe form it consists of a stiffness of the body, with slow shuffling gait and retropulsion on turns; weakness of oropharyngeal muscles (**pseudobulbar palsy**), with drooling, difficulty in swallowing, and dysarthria; and a peculiar behavioral syndrome called **emotional lability**. In this condition there is a dissociation of the sensation or experience of mood and affect from the ability to express mood and affect. Facial expressions and bodily attitudes of happiness or, more commonly, grief, appear and disappear without the active, voluntary control of the patient and without regard for the actual mood of the patient at the time.

Subcortical hemorrhagic or ischemic infarctions also may be small or moderate in size. In such cases one generally expects good recovery from the consequent subcortical aphasia. Ironically, hemorrhagic infarctions, which are often considered more serious than ischemic infarctions (because hemorrhage seems more often to lead to death in the early states), may yield better long-term results in aphasia if the patient survives. This is because hemorrhage tends to dissect its way between the brain cells, leaving many neurons temporarily but not permanently disabled, whereas occlusive ischemia destroys all cells deprived of oxygen.

A stroke that causes aphasia and hemiplegia, as bad as that may be, may distract the clinician from a potentially more serious medical problem: cardiovascular disease. Most middle-aged, hypertensive patients who have atherosclerosis-related strokes have heart disease. As many as 25% of them have already had previous heart attacks, recognized or silent. It is usually the heart disease, not the stroke, that will affect long-term medical prognosis. A significant percentage of these newly aphasic patients will have another (or a first) heart attack, often fatal, within the next 5 years after the aphasia-producing stroke.

This is especially true if the patient is diabetic. One of the effects of diabetes is a speeding up of the process of atherosclerosis. An obese, diabetic, hypertensive person who does not exercise much is at high risk for stroke and heart attack. Smoking compounds the problem, as it can narrow blood vessels and contribute independently to cerebrovascular and cardiovascular disease. Some speech-language pathologists may think it is not within their realm of responsibility to advise persons with aphasia about medical issues. Although this reluctance is understandable, treating aphasia means treating a whole person, not just a specific disability.

II. Traumatic Brain Injury

Second only to stroke, traumatic brain injury (TBI) is the next most common cause of sudden-onset aphasia. There are more than 450,000 cases of closed head injury requiring hospitalization each year. As many as one third of these patients have some sort of speech or language disorder. Unfortunately, as yet there is no accurate breakdown of figures to indicate how many of these disorders are aphasic or dysarthric or related to mutism.

Understanding pathophysiologic mechanisms of head injury that underlie neurobehavioral disorders can facilitate development of a treatment plan. The following description is simplified and highly schematic. One may consider head injury to affect the brain in two ways: (a) focally and (b) multifocally or diffusely.

Focal damage to the brain occurs directly under the point of impact (the **coup injury**) and in a direct line on the opposite side of the brain, as the brain is thrust against the inner table of the skull (the **contrecoup injury**). At these points the brain may suffer a **contusion** (bruise) on the cortical surface. Deeper within the brain under the point of impact there may be a **traumatic intracerebral hemorrhage**. Aphasic or other cognitive deficits may emerge, depending on the location of the contusion. The most common aphasic syndrome seen after closed head injury is anomic aphasia. Other aphasic syndromes also occur, although conduction aphasia is decidedly uncommon.

Focal damage to the brain also occurs in another way. When the head suffers an acceleration-deceleration injury, the brain moves within the cranial vault. This movement causes contusions and abrasions in preferential locations: the frontal poles, the temporal tips, the undersurface of the frontal lobes (orbitofrontal), the undersurface of the temporal lobes, and occasionally the occipital poles. This brain damage causes a range of altered behaviors that can influence aphasia; chief among them is **frontal-lobe syndrome**. Called by Geschwind a syndrome of "irritable euphoric apathy," patients with this behavioral disturbance may exhibit lack of interest punctuated by occasional outbursts of irritability and inappropriate jocularity. Markedly reduced insight and impoverished ability to plan for the future are additional features of this syndrome.

The brain is also affected in a diffuse, or less focal, manner with traumatic brain injury. Sudden severe trauma to the head can cause rupture of white matter sheaths protecting the axons coursing to and from the cortex, and even rupture the axons themselves. Although this phenomenon, called **diffuse axonal injury (DAI)**, occurs throughout the cerebral hemispheres and brain stem, it is most prominent in the frontal lobes, compounding the problems caused by frontal pole and orbitofrontal contusions. Added to the signs and symptoms described above may be perseveration and fluctuations in level of alertness.

In addition to the damage caused directly to the brain by the impact of the injury, secondary effects on brain function result from vascular disruption. Hemorrhage may occur between the dura and the arachnoid membrane, causing a **subdural hematoma**, or between the arachnoid membrane and the brain, causing a **subarachnoid hemorrhage**.

Subdural hematomas occur with increasing frequency with aging and are common in persons with abnormalities of blood clotting, such as alcoholics or persons receiving anticoagulants. Decreased level of consciousness is an early finding, followed by progressive unilateral hemispheric signs and evidence of brain stem dysfunction. We have seen a small number of patients with left parietotemporal subdural hematoma and underlying contusion whose presenting sign was aphasia. Evacuation of the hematoma in two of these cases resulted in rapid resolution of the aphasic syndrome.

Subarachnoid hemorrhage may result from head injury, although another common cause is rupture of an aneurysm. An acute subarachnoid hemorrhage usually begins with a sudden, unusually severe headache, often described by the patient as if an external object smacked against the head with great force. Except for transient dizziness or brief, transient loss of consciousness, there may be no other obvious symptoms beyond the persistent severe headache, often located at the back of the neck. Signs of subarachnoid hemorrhage may be graded from mild to severe for purposes of determining prognosis. In the mild form the patient may have slight neck stiffness (due to blood irritating the meninges) but no other neurological findings. In the most severe form patients may progress rapidly from drowsiness to stupor to deep coma, with decerebrate rigidity (exaggerated posture, with continuous spasm of muscles, especially the extensor muscles).

When bleeding has occurred in the subarachnoid space, there is a risk of development of fibrous adhesions, which may interfere with the normal flow and reabsorption of cerebrospinal fluid. Years, months, or even just weeks after a subarachnoid hemorrhage, such impaired reabsorption of cerebrospinal fluid may result in the development of hydrocephalus, with normal pressure when measured by lumbar puncture. This syndrome of **normal pressure**

hydrocephalus (NPH) consists of progressive gait disturbance, urinary incontinence, and signs of frontal system dysfunction. Sometimes only fragments of the syndrome appear rather than the fully developed symptom complex. In such a case, an aphasia therapist may not know why a patient who seems otherwise healthy is not making steady progress in therapy, or may even be deteriorating. Any patient with a prior history of subarachnoid hemorrhage or who has suffered a severe open or closed head injury should be considered a candidate for subsequent development of normal pressure hydrocephalus.

III. Seizures

A seizure is a sudden, transient alteration of neurologic function, often with modification of consciousness, due to an abnormal, excessive, paroxysmal discharge of neurons. There are many possible causes of seizures: brain tumor, brain scarring from head injury, infection of the brain, embolic infarction, metabolic dysfunction, and so forth. **Epilepsy** is a neurologic disorder manifested by recurrent seizures. The following lists delineate the different seizure types:

Generalized Seizures

1. Absence (petit mal)

2. Major motor (grand mal, tonic-clonic)

3. Myoclonic

4. Infantile spasms

5. Febrile

Partial Seizures (Focal Seizures)

1. Simple (primary focal)

   (a) Motor

   (b) Sensory

   (c) Autonomic

2. Complex (psychomotor, temporo-limbic)

   (a) Psychic/cognitive/affective

   (b) Automatisms

Descriptions of these seizure types (with the exception of myoclonic, infantile, and febrile) follow in sections A. and B.

A seizure can have several different components, any one of which can be relevant to aphasia. The **aura** is the first stage of a seizure associated with electroencephalographic changes. This may be the only portion of a seizure that a patient can recall. The aura occurs in partial, not in generalized, seizures resulting from a localizable or focal lesion. Often the focus of the brain abnormality will announce itself by specific signs or symptoms during the aura. For example, the sensation of an unpleasant odor may point to a lesion in the uncinate cortex; flashing lights, to a lesion in the visual cortex; speech output disturbance, to a lesion in the temporal lobe.

The **ictus** is the main part of a seizure and has a duration of a few seconds to several minutes, depending on the seizure type. The ictus begins suddenly, and the patient usually has no recollection of this part of the event.

The **postictal stage** is that part of the seizure in which the patient begins to recover. Brain function is often abnormal in this stage, and the patient may be drowsy and confused, usually for about 15–30 minutes but sometimes for hours. In **absence attacks** (see A. "Generalized Seizures"), however, alertness may return immediately after the ictus.

The **interictal period** is the period between seizures. **Status epilepticus** is a condition in which there is no interictal period. That is, each subsequent seizure begins during the postictal period of the preceding seizure. This may be a life-threatening situation. Some patients with epilepsy may be entirely normal during the interictal period; others may show increasing changes in personality.

A. Generalized Seizures

Absence attacks, also called **petit mal epilepsy**, usually occur in childhood, persisting commonly into the teens but rarely into adulthood. The spells begin with an abrupt loss of awareness of what is happening, lasting just a few seconds. During the spell the patient may have a bewildered or blank look on his or her face, but a person in the patient's immediate vicinity may not know that anything is wrong. These attacks may occur dozens or scores of times during a day. A child in school, for example, may repeatedly miss a key word or two in several sections of an important lesson. Following the attack the child picks up the thread of the presentation, occasionally without realizing that anything has been lost. Neither is the teacher necessarily aware that there is anything wrong, except that "the child doesn't always seem to be paying attention and is performing poorly on tests." A clinician examining a patient with such spells may confirm the suspicion by asking the patient from time to time to repeat precisely what has just been said. Patients with ongoing, frequent, untreated absence attacks will perform the task normally except for a blank period, reflecting the momentary lapse of awareness.

Often patients with petit mal epilepsy will have no abnormal movements. Some, however, have a transient drooping of the head, blinking of the eyes, or other brief, repetitive, automatic movement. A characteristic electroencephalographic pattern is found: from a normal pattern, the EEG abruptly shows a repeating pattern of spike and wave occurring three times per second during the attack (called the "3 per second spike and wave pattern"), reverting to normal as the spell ends.

Adults may also have such spells, often with a different EEG pattern. When these attacks occur in children, usually no underlying cerebral lesion is found. When they occur in adults, often a seizure focus is discovered in the temporal lobe. It is easy to see how such a disorder, if it continues unrecognized and untreated, could interfere with progress in aphasia therapy.

The syndrome of **major motor seizures**, also called **grand mal epilepsy**, **tonic-clonic seizures**, or **primary generalized seizures**, is manifested by recurrent episodes of sudden loss of consciousness, with associated motor activity (such as collapsing to the ground with violent shaking of the muscles; i.e., the convulsion or tonic-clonic activity), a brief shriek at the moment of unconsciousness as air is forced through the adducted vocal cords, and involuntary urinary or fecal incontinence. The rate of convulsive jerking (stiffening and relaxing) decreases during the first 2–3 minutes, and finally the patient lies limp, remaining unconscious for another minute or two. Gradually consciousness returns, with a period of postictal confusion, fatigue, weakness, and, sometimes, headache, all of variable duration.

When these patients are flung to the ground, as if gripped by external forces, they may suffer serious injury—tongue biting, head injury, or broken vertebra, with blood drooling or frothing at the lips. For the layperson who has never witnessed a convulsive seizure, these attacks can be quite frightening. (Some of the so-called "witches" of Salem, thought to be possessed by the devil, were women with grand mal epilepsy.) If an attack occurs, stay calm; it will usually stop within a few minutes. Protect the patient from injury. Do not stick a spoon, your finger, or anything hard into the patient's mouth. Turn the patient onto one side to prevent aspiration and place his or her head on soft padding to prevent head injury. Do not restrain the person or try to control the shaking.

During an attack the electroencephalogram has a characteristic pattern: high voltage, generalized spike discharges. Considerable muscle artefact is seen on the EEG during an attack. In the postictal stage the EEG pattern generally consists of widespread, relatively low-voltage slowing. During the interictal period the EEG may be normal.

Epilepsy should always be a clinical consideration if a patient who had an aphasia-producing stroke is not making expected progress in therapy months after the stroke. Epilepsy may be "subclinical." That is, there is abnormal spike discharge activity on the EEG, reflecting abnormal brain electrical activity, but there may be no overt seizure. The abnormal brain electrical activity may be adversely affecting recovery from aphasia, even though no convulsions are evident. As many as 25% of the patients with stroke affecting cerebral cortex may develop a seizure disorder, usually from 6–9 months after the stroke.

B. Partial Seizures

Partial seizures, also called **focal epilepsy**, may be simple or complex. Simple focal seizures may involve motor system or sensory system or autonomic system. Complex focal epilepsies may include all three of these systems, and an affective and cognitive component as well; this cluster of features occurs in the syndrome of temporal lobe or **temporo-limbic epilepsy (TLE)**, discussed further below. Partial seizures may be caused by any disease or injury that can affect the brain locally, such as stroke, brain tumor, head injury, intracerebral abcess, vascular malformation, a patch of localized encephalitis, and so forth.

Simple focal seizures are caused by highly localized, focal lesions. If the lesion is in the motor system, for example, the seizure may consist of a rhythmic movement of a finger or hand, toe or foot, or other body part. At times a focal seizure will start distally in a limb, as in a finger for instance, and spread over the course of several minutes to involve the rest of the limb, then to include one whole side of the body in the rhythmic shaking activity, without loss of consciousness. This phenomenon is called a **jacksonian march** (after Hughlings Jackson, who provided early and vivid descriptions).

Simple focal seizures also may affect the sensory system, involving selected parts of the body. The patient with such a disorder would complain, for example, of recurrent episodes of numbness or tingling in one limb. Recurrent episodes of flashing lights occurring in one visual hemifield or spells of visual hallucinations may reflect seizure activity emanating from visual cortical cells.

Sections of the temporal lobe are particularly epileptogenic; that is, lesions in these sections of the brain are more likely to provoke seizures than lesions in, say, the parietal lobe. Lesions within the zone of language, especially in the temporal lobe, may cause the syndrome of **paroxysmal aphasia**. This clinical phenomenon falls somewhere between the categories of simple and complex partial epilepsy. The features consist, typically, of speech blocking and word-finding pauses characteristic of certain varieties of anomic aphasia. Not infrequently there is an associated transient confusional state, which may produce impairment of auditory comprehension. The French neurologist Henry Hécaen used to say that paroxysmal aphasia was a common presenting sign of malignant tumor in the left temporal lobe. That has been our experience as well, although any of the causes of focal epilepsy could produce paroxysmal aphasia.

Temporo-limbic epilepsy (TLE), also called **complex partial epilepsy** or **psychomotor epilepsy**, is a syndrome manifested by recurrent episodes of involuntary, apparently purposeful, complex motor activity carried out in a repetitive manner, such as pacing or opening and closing a drawer, with associated psychic phenomena and amnesia for the event. The associated phenomena may consist of memory aberrations, such as **déjà vu** (a sense of having seen or experienced an event before), hallucinations within any sensory modality, feelings of paranoia, and affective changes. Repetitive movements of a somewhat less complex nature, such as lip smacking or jaw movements, called **automatisms**, are frequent. Spells of TLE often are preceded by an aura that may be vegetative (e.g., nausea, vertigo), sensory (e.g., unpleasant odors), or affective (e.g., a sense of fear, dread, or anger).

Considerable attention has been paid to the question of the interictal personality of patients with temporo-limbic epilepsy. Although it seems likely that the majority of patients with TLE do not have interictal personality disorders, some do. In the milder versions there is a cluster of symptoms and signs: hypergraphia, tangentiality in conversations, decreased sexual interest, hyperreligiosity, a sense that the patient has been placed on earth to accomplish a significant mission of universal importance, and a poorly described phenomenon called "stickiness" or viscosity, in which the patient has a tendency to cling (verbally) to a listener. In the more severe forms there is a psychotic disorder that has been called schizophreniform, to suggest that it shares features with classical schizophrenic psychosis but with differences.

IV. Tumors

Tumors of the nervous system may arise from within the brain itself, as with **gliomas** (the most malignant of which is called **glioblastoma**), from tissues near the brain that can impinge on brain substance, such as with **meningiomas**, or from regions of the body distant from the brain but that send metastatic cells either to the substance of the brain, such as with metastatic lung or breast cancer, or to tissues near the brain.

Symptoms of aphasia may appear in different patterns depending on the type of tumor, its location, and the rate of growth. A slowly growing glioma in the temporal lobe, for example, may manifest itself as a mild and slowly progressive anomia for years before anyone thinks to look for a tumor. This is especially true because word-finding difficulties are common language features of normal aging, and tumors are more common in older than in younger adults. Paroxysmal aphasia, as discussed in the preceding section on seizures, may be the first sign of a primary or metastatic tumor in the temporal lobe. A tumor that spares the zone of language altogether may still influence language function in aphasia by causing increased intracranial pressure. In such a case, anomia, nonaphasic misnaming, drowsiness, and a mild confusional state may all be seen.

The ethical question of whether to treat a patient with aphasia due to a malignant intracerebral tumor is not easy to answer, and a decision must be made in each case individually. More than half of all intracranial tumors are malignant, with poor prognosis. On one side is the desire of the clinician to help the patient in any way possible, to keep hope alive and to maintain or improve quality of life in the remaining months. On the other is the relentless progression of the lesion interfering with gains from therapy, and the burning contemporary bioethical issue of who should receive medical care in an era of limited, and even declining, resources and increasing need. Our society is living longer, thereby increasing the numbers of patients still surviving with stroke, tumor, and now dementia. These ethical questions will increase in prominence in coming years.

V. Dementia

Dementia is a clinical syndrome manifested by progressive deterioration of cognitive function, changes in personality and behavior, and impairment of social and psychosocial adaptation. In the past 15 years, considerable research has been carried out in the related fields of dementia, language in normal aging, language in dementia, and aphasia in dementia. Of particular interest to the aphasia therapist are dementia of the Alzheimer's type, multi-infarct dementia, and Pick's disease.

No adequate evaluation of aphasia in dementia can be carried out without some knowledge of the language changes in normal aging. As people get older changes occur in language of a characteristic and predictable nature. Word-finding difficulty (anomia) develops, slowly at first, but then more rapidly after age 70. This naming disorder is due to a combination of factors, including progressive perceptual problems, increasing impairment of processing efficiency, deficits in lexical access, and disorder of semantic memory. Older people develop dysfluencies in output (e.g., hesitancies) but at the same time may produce more output, and more linguistically elaborate output, without necessarily adding more themes or meaning to their words. Mild auditory comprehension deficits develop, partially though not entirely due to auditory perceptual deficits.

A. Alzheimer's Disease

Alzheimer's disease is the most common form of dementia. The diagnosis can only be made with certainty by neuropathological study, demonstrating decreasing numbers of cortical neurons and abundant senile plaques, neurofibrillary degeneration of neurons (tangles), granulovacuolar degeneration, and increased accumulation of lipofucsin. In our opinion these neuropathological changes represent a final common pathway resulting from several or many different etiological origins; and Alzheimer's disease should be considered a group of different illnesses with overlapping clinical features and common neuropathological findings (although this clinical presumption has yet to be proven).

Clinically we have seen at least two major variants. In the common form, the symptoms start with memory disorder, language dysfunction (anomia and subsequently auditory comprehension impairment), and visuospatial disability, all suggestive of parieto-temporal disease. Eventually, signs of frontal system dysfunction appear (see description in preceding section on head injury). Aphasia and apraxia are common. The aphasia develops in stages, resembling classical patterns of anomic, then transcortical sensory, then Wernicke's aphasia, although other features of dementia are virtually always present as well. We have never seen severe speech output disorders or nonfluent aphasia in the early stages of typical Alzheimer's disease. If signs of anterior aphasia occur early in a dementing illness, the clinician should assume that the dementing illness is other than Alzheimer's disease. The second variant starts with frontal signs, with the posterior cortical features appearing later.

B. Pick's Disease

Pick's disease is a dementing illness in which cerebral atrophy occurs selectively in specific lobes of the brain, frontal and temporal, and thus is also called **Pick's lobar atrophy**. Neuropathological confirmation of this illness is provided by the presence of **Pick's cells** (swollen nerve cells with silver staining inclusions) not typical of Alzheimer's disease. From an aphasiological point of view, the neuropathology of Pick's disease is particularly interesting because the posterior portion of the superior temporal gyrus (i.e., Wernicke's area) typically is spared. Thus, the patterns of language disorder are different in these two dementing illnesses. The language disorder in Pick's disease often starts with signs of motor-speech impairment, unlike that seen in Alzheimer's disease. Another common characteristic of the aphasia of Pick's disease is the striking loss of

abstract attitude, and with it the loss of the ability to cate-
gorize, to find superordinates, to find similarities, or to find
multiple uses for a single word. Otherwise, the clinical features
of the two syndromes have considerable overlap, although, of
course, Pick's disease always starts with frontal lobe signs,
whereas Alzheimer's usually starts with posterior cortical signs.

C. Multi-infarct Dementia

Multiple strokes are a relatively less common cause of dementia. The lacunar state, described previously, is one of the neurobehavioral syndromes associated with strokes. A true multi-
infarct dementia (MID) is probably the result of a combination
of several large strokes affecting cortical and subcortical tissue
together with small lacunar strokes in deep white matter of the
frontal lobes and in basal ganglia. Patterns of aphasia will
vary, depending on size and location of strokes. This cause of
dementia is probably much less common than it is given credit
for. Generally one is taught that a distinguishing feature of
multi-infarct dementia from Alzheimer's disease is the step-
wise development of neurologic signs in MID. We have seen not
a few cases, however, in which presumed multi-infarct dementia developed insidiously and progressively, and presumed
Alzheimer's disease developed in a step-wise fashion. To our
minds the issue of the nature and frequency of occurrence of
multi-infarct dementia is still an open question.

Selected Readings

Adams, R., & Victor, M. (1989). *Principles of neurology* (4th ed.). New York: McGraw-Hill.

Caplan, L., & Stein, R. (1986). *Stroke: A clinical approach.* Boston: Butterworth.

Weisberg, L., Strub, R., & Garcia, C. (1989). *Essentials of clinical neurology* (2nd ed.). Rockville, MD: Aspen.

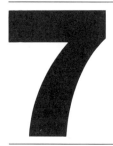

Neuropsychological Examination: The Process Approach

Roberta Gallagher, Ph.D.

Clinical neuropsychology is an applied discipline that seeks to integrate knowledge of brain-behavior relationships gleaned from the fields of neurology and experimental psychology with precise and comprehensive test procedures developed from the clinical psychology tradition. Philosophical differences guide the various traditions of neuropsychological evaluation as practiced today. Two approaches in particular are popular and can be contrasted. The quantitative psychometric approach stresses a fixed, standardized test battery, with cutoff scores on each test reflecting cerebral pathology. The pattern of deficits leads to "actuarial" conclusions about the presence, lateralization, and localization of brain damage. In contemporary medical settings, however, neuroimaging by computed tomography (CT) and magnetic resonance imaging (MRI) are routinely available, and the anatomy of the lesion is often well documented before the patient is referred for neuropsychological evaluation.

The **process approach** to neuropsychological assessment, pioneered by Edith Kaplan more than 20 years ago, developed from the conviction that reliance on test scores often obscures critical information about individual differences in cognitive styles and strategies, preserved abilities, and the way in which a task was passed or failed. This information is useful in developing an understanding of a patient's abilities, how any weaknesses might best be supported and compensated for, and how cognitive strengths might be capitalized upon in therapeutic interventions.

The process approach does not reject quantitative, standardized tests and in fact utilizes them to provide a point of reference both to an individual's relative performance under standardized circumstances and to that individual's own subsequent performance over time. The process approach, however, seeks to expand the utility of such tests by structuring the evaluation as a dynamic relationship between examiner and patient. On-line changes by the examiner in task parameters and careful documentation of the patient's exact behavior are considered more valuable diagnostically than the tests scores alone. If limit testing, probing, and changing the task requirements are carried out after the item has been presented and scored according to standardized administration, then the examiner may obtain not only valid standardized scores but also a wealth of additional and highly individualized information.

I. The Neuropsychological Evaluation of the Aphasic Patient

Neuropsychological evaluation of an aphasic patient provides a comprehensive profile of current cognitive and affective status that helps both patient and family understand and adjust to changes in function and provides information critical to treatment planning. Regardless of the theoretical orientation of the clinical neuropsychologist, a wide range of cognitive functions are assessed, including the following:

1. Affective state and motivation

2. Orientation

3. Ability to establish and sustain a focus of attention

4. Language

5. Visuospatial organization

6. Ability to learn and retain new information and to access previously learned material

7. Ability to plan and execute complex tasks

A. History

A thorough examination begins with a careful medical history. Because many aphasic individuals are unable to provide such information themselves, contact with a reliable family member and a review of the medical records are important. Age, time since onset of aphasia, type and extent of lesion, and handedness are all significant factors in recovery and are necessary for placing a test performance in its appropriate context. In addition, it is helpful to obtain as much information as possible about the individual's premorbid intelligence and adaptive functioning as well as about any preexisting deficits, such as a developmental learning disability. The patient's educational and employment history are often a good index of the premorbid level of functioning, but these of course may be limited by socioeconomic constraints even in very bright and capable individuals.

B. Behavioral Observations

Assessment of the patient's motivation and personal investment in doing well on the testing is necessary for interpreting the results. The examiner may not always feel that the data accurately represent the patient's level of performance. For example, if the patient is trying especially hard to please the examiner and the setting is highly structured, the patient realistically may not function at that level on a consistent basis in the everyday environment. On the other hand, if a patient is upset, depressed, or resistant to being tested, these observations should be noted and the test data interpreted accordingly. It may be sufficient to evaluate the patient's behavior and affect informally through direct questioning and observation over the course of testing, or a more structured diagnostic interview of the patient and family may be necessary if there is evidence of significant psychopathology.

It is important to note whether the patient is aware of and/or discouraged by failures on tasks, how frustration is handled, and whether interactions with the examiner are socially appropriate. Aphasic patients may be unable to verbalize their feelings, and changes in innervation of facial musculature may render it difficult to interpret facial affect. Moreover, in the presence of bilateral white matter damage, there may be disinhibition of superficial displays of affect that do not reflect the patient's mood state. It is important for all clinicians working with brain-damaged patients to be sensitive to the issues of affective and behavioral changes (see chapter 20). Typically the therapist spends much more time with the patient than the primary physician and thus is in a position to observe a broader sample of behavior that might otherwise have gone unreported and untreated.

The examiner must remain sensitive to the subject's mood, ability to work before becoming fatigued, tendency to perseverate, and motivation throughout the course of testing. These factors not only may influence the validity of the test results but also will bear on formulating an interdisciplinary treatment plan and structuring therapies. In choosing a test battery, one must take into account the wide range of impairments and spared abilities that may occur throughout the spectrum of aphasia, and flexibility is called for in administering and interpreting tests.

C. Overview of Areas of Cognition Evaluated

1. **Attention/concentration.** Observation over the course of the evaluation will establish whether the patient was consistently wide awake, alert, and able to establish and sustain a focus of attention, all of which are basic to reliable testing. Distractibility by external or internal stimuli should be noted. Vigilance can be assessed by a continuous performance task, which may consist simply of the examiner reading random letters aloud at a fixed rate and having the subject respond by raising a hand when one designated letter is heard. A visual analogue of this task can consist of presenting the letters serially on a computer screen, in which case the subject presses a button when the target appears. The task can be made more complex by specifying that the target letter is responded to only if it is preceded by another designated letter (e.g., the subject is to respond to the letter *o* only when it has been preceded immediately by an *x*). This task is useful in determining not only the level of attention, but also whether attention decreases as the task progresses over the course of a few minutes due to fatigue or distractibility.

Decreased span of attention, or the amount of information one can consciously keep in mind at one time, is a limiting factor in working with many brain-damaged individuals. This ability is tapped on both the *Wechsler Adult Intelligence Scale–Revised* (WAIS-R; Wechsler, 1981) and the *Wechsler Memory Scale–Revised* (WMS-R; Wechsler, 1986) by having the subject repeat or reverse strings of digits spoken by the examiner. With aphasic patients, however, assessment of auditory verbal span may be impractical because of auditory comprehension and verbal production problems. Even attempting to have the individual point to the digits on a number card may not be feasible because some patients may point to one number but be unable to inhibit saying a different one, so that their intended response is difficult to ascertain. The WMS-R contains a nonverbal pointing span subtest in which the examiner points sequentially to certain squares from a random array, and the subject must point to them in the same order (or in the *reverse* order on a subsequent condition of the task).

2. **Language/verbal abilities.** A standard neuropsychological evaluation typically screens a wide range of language abilities, including fluency, articulation, word retrieval, comprehension, repetition, reading, and writing. When the subject of the evaluation already has been identified as aphasic and is being seen concurrently by a speech-language pathologist, any language testing planned in the course of the neuropsychological evaluation should be coordinated to ensure that it is not redundant. In any case it is important to note how communication abilities may have influenced the individual's test results. For example, poor performance on a particular task may result from impaired comprehension of test instructions, or an individual may know the information when verbal responses are required but be unable to express the information adequately.

Whenever possible, the WAIS-R Verbal scale is administered to tap language abilities, but in most cases the aphasic patient's communication problems render this unfeasible or yield invalid results. The Information subtest of the WAIS-R taps the subject's fund of general, previously acquired semantic knowledge. Unlike many of the other verbal subtests, the answers to the Information questions are brief and specific (e.g., "What is the capital of Italy?"), so that at times they may be answered by individuals who have difficulty formulating the lengthy explanations or definitions called for by the other subtests. For those persons for whom even brief verbal responses are impossible, Kaplan, Fein, Morris, and Delis (in press) have developed a multiple-choice form of the Information subtest. The choices are printed on laminated cards, which the examiner shows to the subject while reading each option. The *Goodglass Number Information Test,* a series of 24 items dealing with familiar numerical facts (e.g., "How many cards are there in a deck?"), is another test given to tap a category of semantic information. Depending on the patient's abilities, the format may be either free recall or multiple choice.

Although use of multiple-choice answers in these situations may provide the most reliable estimate of preserved general knowledge, the method is not without problems. A multiple-choice format may inflate an individual's score, as *recognition* of information is generally easier than *retrieval.* This consideration is particularly important for a person who not only is aphasic but who also has a deficit in accessing information stored in memory. Moreover, multiple choice can be problematic for some individuals with frontal lobe involvement; these patients may have difficulty carrying out the series of comparisons and contrasts necessary to evaluate the appropriateness of each response relative to the others. Such persons may impulsively choose the first foil that bears some relation to the target response and then be unable to disengage from that response. Other patients show a response bias, seeming "pulled" to select the response occupying a given serial position, such as the first or the last item presented.

3. **Visuoperceptual/constructional abilities.** It is usually possible to administer the WAIS-R Performance scale to aphasic patients, although it may be necessary at times to depart from the strict standards of administration. Because of problems in auditory comprehension and/or establishing response set, the examiner may find it necessary to repeat and further explain the instructions, even modeling the desired response and helping the subject through an unscored practice item that is similar in content to the test items. Care must be exercised to keep the stimuli in the patient's intact visual field if there are problems with hemianopsia or visual neglect. Further, many aphasic patients are hemiplegic and thus must use their nondominant hand to complete these and other tasks, and this disadvantage must be considered in evaluating test performances.

Several of the WAIS-R Performance scale subtests are timed, with cutoff time limits and with extra credit for rapid performance. The standardized scale scores only credit work that has been completed within these time limits. It is useful to note the patient's performance as of the cutoff time but to allow additional time as necessary to finish the task, assuming that the patient is continuing to work toward a solution and is not overwhelmed or extremely frustrated. Then, in addition to the calculation of the scale score according to the manual's guidelines, a separate score can be calculated based on correct responses without regard to time limits.

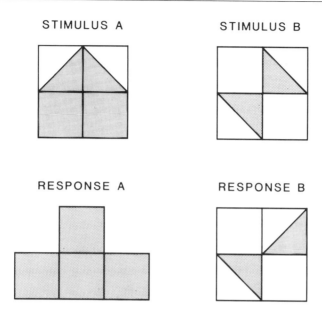

STIMULUS A   STIMULUS B

RESPONSE A   RESPONSE B

FIG. 7.1. The error in Response A violates the basic 2 x 2 matrix. In Response B the matrix is preserved, but an error of detail occurs in the upper right quadrant.

A rule of thumb in interpreting the WAIS-R is that deficits in the Verbal and Performance scales are associated with damage to the left and right cerebral hemispheres, respectively. A difference between the two scales of 15 points is both statistically and clinically significant, and is suggestive of lateralized cerebral pathology. Most aphasic individuals, however, manifest some impairment on the Performance scale subtests relative to their estimated premorbid level of competence. Nevertheless, their errors typically will differ *qualitatively* from those of right-hemisphere-damaged patients (Kaplan, 1988). For example, right-hemisphere-damaged patients frequently fail to appreciate the basic 2×2 or 3×3 design matrix required to complete the Block Design task, so that their errors contain gross distortions of the gestalt (see Fig. 7.1). In contrast, the intact right hemisphere usually ensures that this matrix is preserved when left-hemisphere-damaged individuals perform the task; their errors tend to be ones in which internal details of the design are incorrect.

The WAIS-R Digit Symbol subtest, in which the patient must utilize psychomotor energy in rapidly transcribing a

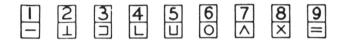

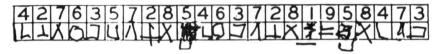

FIG. 7.2. In attempting to copy the symbols corresponding to the numbers in the key, this subject at times was unable to inhibit copying the number itself. Note the monitoring and attempts to correct the errors.

code, usually must be omitted from calculating Performance IQ in aphasic patients because they often are using the nondominant or a weakened dominant hand, and thus their slow, laborious output is penalized unfairly. This task is of interest, however, insofar as it can provide clues about perseveration and pull to the perceptual features of test stimuli when the coded symbols are examined individually. For example, in Fig. 7.2 it is clear that the patient has incorporated visual elements of the numeral "5" into the symbol that stands for the "5." This patient consistently self-monitored and self-corrected the response but was unable to inhibit it each time.

In another frequently seen type of error, the subject might, after coding the symbol for "3," be pulled to seek the next "4" and then the next "5" rather than dealing with the next digit in the random series.

Visuospatial functions are assessed additionally by several subtests from the *Boston Spatial-Quantitative Battery* (Goodglass & Kaplan, 1983), including a series of drawings to command and to copy. The former provides information about the subject's ability to visualize and execute a representation of an object in its absence, and the latter provides information on the subject's ability to attend to details and reproduce accurately. Examples of the objects include the following: a clock set for 10 after 11, which demands symmetry, ability to represent numbers, and ability to conceptualize where the hands should be placed as well as resistance to impulsively placing the hands on

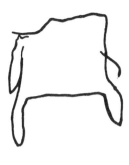
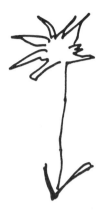

FIG. 7.3. An elephant (left) and a flower (right), drawn to command by aphasic patients, show attention to outer contours but minimal internal details.

the numerals 10 and 11; and a cube, which calls for ability to represent a sense of three-dimensional perspective. The drawing tasks also are helpful in providing information about hemispatial neglect, graphomotor skill, part/whole integration, and planning. In Fig. 7.3, examples of drawings by aphasic patients illustrate the tendency of individuals with left-hemisphere lesions to focus on the outer contours of a drawing while neglecting internal details.

As noted, on these and other graphomotor tasks, hemiplegic subjects who must use their nondominant hand would be expected to show some clumsiness, as would most normal individuals constrained from using their preferred hand. Hemiplegic patients may be unable to anchor the paper with the opposite hand in a normal manner, a problem that can be alleviated either by securing the paper to the desk with removable tape or by providing a clipboard.

4. **Learning/memory.** Informal observation provides some pertinent information about **anterograde memory**, or the individual's ability to form and preserve new memories. In an inpatient setting, the patient's orientation to the surroundings and to the hospital staff is important to note, as is the ability to remember the location of his or her room, the lounge, the nursing station, and so forth. The patient who is able to arrive at the testing office unassisted at the appointed time has revealed a great deal about memory,

motivation, and adaptive capabilities. Comprehensive assessment of learning and memory requires consideration of both verbal and nonverbal modalities and compares the ability to learn and retain new information with retention of and effective access to previously acquired knowledge. Often neglected in formal memory testing is **procedural learning**, or the capacity to acquire motor skills and the mastery of concrete tasks, even in the absence of any conscious awareness on the part of the subject of having learned the tasks. Procedural learning may be spared even in the presence of severe deficits in memory for the type of facts and data commonly tested, and such preserved abilities can be extremely important in practical rehabilitative programs.

Formal testing of aphasic individuals using the WMS-R may have to rely heavily on the nonverbal subtests, which include reproduction of visual designs, nonverbal paired associate learning (in which a color and a nonrepresentational figure are paired), "figural memory" (multiple-choice recognition of previously presented designs), and nonverbal pointing span. With the exception of the reproduction of designs, the nonverbal subtests require only pointing responses, and so do not unduly reflect difficulties with graphomotor production.

Again, deviation from the standard administration is often called for when using the WMS-R with an aphasic individual. When reproductions of visual designs are executed poorly, one can probe the responses with multiple-choice and matching conditions after the immediate recall condition. This modification technically confounds calculation of the delayed memory index, but the advantages of the additional qualitative information generally offset this problem. The immediate and delayed recall probes can be compared informally in this modification.

It is very often infeasible to administer the attentional and verbal subtests of the WMS-R to aphasic individuals. A multiple-choice probe of the logical memory stories can be administered both immediately and after a 30-minute filled delay. Any errors committed in the initial recall trial are corrected immediately by the examiner. This procedure reveals whether newly learned verbal information has been retained after a delay. Providing feedback shows in some cases that a long narrative overwhelms the patient's ability to grasp its content effectively and that the patient's learning and retention have been facilitated by breaking the material down into more manageable units.

5. **Executive functions.** Planning, organizational, and goal-directed behaviors may be described as indices of **executive functioning**. Most basic is the ability to establish response set, or to ascertain the nature of the task and respond accordingly. Even when they are able to comprehend what is being requested, some patients are unable to organize and execute their responses in conformance with the request. Others initially achieve the correct form of responding but are unable to retain the task requirements over time. In such cases, the subject may have become distracted by some other external or internal stimulus, or a competing response may have contaminated the target behavior. Some tasks explicitly call for alternation of response programs to test whether interference will take place. For example, the examiner may ask the subject to hold up two fingers each time the examiner holds up one, and vice versa. If this is carried out successfully, the task may be modified to determine whether the subject can shift flexibly to a new set of requirements without interference from the previous motor program. Susceptibility to this type of interference from previous stimuli is known as **perseveration** and is discussed in the following section. Additional measures of ability to shift between ongoing motor patterns include having the patient write a continuous line of the cursively written letters *mnmnmn*, and/or similar alternating and repeating graphomotor tasks, and repetition of a three-step manual sequence as suggested by Luria (1973). Poor performance on these tasks can be probed further by providing the patient with a verbal strategy (e.g., suggesting a descriptive name for each hand position, such as "knock, slap, chop") to see whether the patient can incorporate this and profit from it behaviorally.

Executive abilities also include one's approach to complex tasks. Thus, even on tasks that have other explicit diagnostic goals, it is important to assess whether the patient planned and executed the task in a logical, systematic manner or approached it haphazardly. For example, a complex graphomotor task that may be aimed primarily at assessing visuospatial abilities can reveal a great deal about the individual's organizational strategies and planning skills.

Inhibition of irrelevant or counterproductive responses is an executive skill that has a significant impact on an individual's quality of performance across a broad range of cognitive and adaptive tasks. Critical self-monitoring and the ability to self-correct are also crucial to effectively modifying one's own behavior in response to the demands of a complex environment.

6. **Perseveration.** Sandson and Albert (1987) identified three categories of perseveration, each with "its own anatomic, and possibly pharmacologic basis" (p. 1736). The first type is **recurrent** perseveration, in which a previous response recurs to a subsequent stimulus within an ongoing response set. Recurrent perseveration is related to lesions of the left parietal or temporal regions and is the most common type of perseveration encountered in aphasia. The intrusion errors seen in patients with Alzheimer's disease are a delayed form of recurrent perseveration.

The second type of perseveration, called **stuck-in-set**, refers to an inability to shift to a new framework or category and is related to dysfunction of the frontal lobe system, particularly the mesolimbic dopamine projections. A test that is particularly sensitive to stuck-in-set perseveration is the *Wisconsin Card Sorting Test* (Grant & Berg, 1981), in which the subject must match a series of cards to target cards bearing stimuli that vary in color, shape, and number. The target categories are never made explicit but must be deduced by the subject on the basis of the examiner's feedback as to whether a response is right or wrong. Moreover, the target category is changed abruptly after the subject has produced 10 consecutive correct responses. The patient with stuck-in-set perseveration will have difficulty refraining from sorting cards according to a previously reinforced category, despite repeated feedback that these responses are no longer correct.

The third type of perseveration, called **continuous**, refers to instances in which a current behavior is prolonged or continued inappropriately; this is associated with right-hemisphere damage. Continuous perseveration often is observed in graphomotor tasks (e.g., drawing extra loops in copying a multiple-loop design) and may result from difficulty in disengaging one's attention from a stimulus.

II. Frequently Administered Tests

The WAIS-R, WMS-R, and *Coloured Progressive Matrices* are widely used measures in neuropsychological testing that tap a broad array of cognitive abilities. This list is merely representative, however, intended to familiarize the reader with some of the tests that will form the core evaluation within diverse neuropsychological testing orientations. Modifications appropriate to aphasic subjects are included in the discussions of each test. Readers interested in an extensive review of neuropsychological tests and procedures are referred to Lezak (1983).

A. Wechsler Adult Intelligence Scale–Revised

The WAIS-R is the most widely used measure of general cognitive level. It consists of 11 subtests divided between two scales, Verbal and Performance. The WAIS-R yields a Full Scale Intelligence Quotient (IQ) as well as a Verbal and a Performance IQ. Each of these has a mean of 100 and standard deviation of 15. The individual subtests, which each yield a scale score with a mean of 10 and a standard deviation of 3, allow comparison of an individual's performances across the various subtests. Scale scores are based on a comparison of the subject's raw score on a given subtest against a standardization sample of young adults, although computation of the IQ takes age differences into account. Age-corrected scale scores also can be computed, and these are generally more appropriate when characterizing an older aphasic individual's level of performance, particularly when change in status over time is being monitored.

The WAIS-R Verbal scale is made up of the Information, Comprehension, Similarities, Vocabulary, Arithmetic, and Digit Span subtests. The components of the Performance scale are the Picture Completion, Block Design, Object Assembly, Picture Arrangement, and Digit Symbol subtests. Individual subtest scores are highly correlated with the overall IQ in normal individuals, possibly related to a hypothesized general intelligence factor that underlies the structure of the scale. This hypothesized general factor is undermined in the presence of brain damage, and the variability among the subtests is often quite significant. When marked variability occurs, reporting IQ scores is likely to average out the intertest scatter and present an overall index that obscures the individual's strongest and weakest points. It is crucial therefore to highlight specific patterns among the patient's scale scores on the subtests, descriptions of which follow:

1. **Information.** This 29-item test taps the patient's fund of general verbal knowledge and the type of cultural, historical, and scientific knowledge acquired through previous learning. This subtest is highly resistant to the effects of aging and to many types of cerebral insult, and thus in many testing contexts is considered a good index of premorbid functioning. Aphasic individuals, however, often are unable to verbalize this type of knowledge even when it is spared, and therefore a multiple-choice form of the test often is administered.

2. **Comprehension.** These 14 items explore everyday problem solving, ability to apply one's general knowledge to practical situations, and ability to understand the pragmatic meaning of proverbs. Remote memory, understanding of societal conventions, and ability to foresee the consequences of a behavior and to think abstractly are necessary for optimal performance on this subtest.

3. **Similarities.** This measure consists of 13 pairs of objects or concepts (e.g., an orange and a banana). The subject must employ categorical verbal reasoning and concept formation in order to abstract a relevant similarity between the items of a pair. Brain-damaged individuals often have difficulty grasping or retaining the precise task and may have difficulty inhibiting a tendency to respond with a difference rather than a similarity, or to report some salient feature of each item in turn without tying them together. In some cases achievement of the appropriate concept may be facilitated during testing of clinical limits when the task is given additional structure. The examiner might do this by starting a response sentence for the subject, such as "An orange and a banana are *both* . . . ."

4. **Vocabulary.** The 35 items of this subtest evaluate an individual's ability to formulate and express the definitions of

increasingly difficult words. As is the case with the Information subtest, this test correlates very highly with general intelligence and is relatively resistant to many types of cognitive deficits. Vocabulary score, however, is apt to be severely impaired among aphasic individuals. Even the patient who retains some semantic knowledge of a particular word may be unable to retrieve a synonym or organize an adequate definition. According to the scoring guidelines, vague and impoverished responses are penalized. Thus, preserved word knowledge of fluent and nonfluent aphasic patients alike may be markedly underestimated. For this reason one might turn to a multiple-choice test such as the *Peabody Picture Vocabulary Test,* in which the subject must point to the one word from an array of four that best corresponds with a word spoken by the examiner.

5. **Arithmetic.** In this test the examiner orally administers a series of 14 simple arithmetic problems, which the patient then must solve mentally. In addition to calculation ability per se, the structure of this task places significant demands on auditory processing, concentration, ability to manipulate information actively, and ability to disembed the required operations from a "story problem" context. Limit testing may be accomplished on this task by subsequently allowing the patient to read the test items directly and by providing paper and pencil so that calculations can be written. If these measures still fail to elicit the correct response, the story may be eliminated and the task converted to a written calculation.

6. **Digit Span.** The examiner presents a series of random number sequences and the subject must repeat the same numbers in the same order. The sequences become progressively longer and consist of three to nine digits, with two different trials per span until the point at which the subject fails both items. (If errors consist of the correct numbers repeated in the wrong sequence, one can test limits by continuing the task until the subject is unable to repeat the digits even out of sequence.) A backward span is then evaluated by having the subject repeat the digits in reverse order. Nonfluent or paraphasic subjects generally are unable to participate in this task. In such cases an analogue to this task is to present the digits from 1 to 9 on a card and have the patient point to the sequence spoken by the examiner.

7. **Picture Completion.** This subtest features a series of 20 pictures from which some important visual detail is missing. This task requires attention to detail and ability to discriminate truly important missing features from irrelevant or inessential details. Some items can be solved at a simple perceptual level while others require a higher level of abstraction.

8. **Block Design.** The 10 items of this subtest require that the subject analyze and resynthesize a series of two-dimensional figures, which conform to 2×2 or 3×3 matrices, into three-dimensional block constructions. This task requires visuospatial organization and nonverbal problem solving. This task is very sensitive to right-hemisphere damage, but left-hemisphere-damaged individuals also show a decline in performance, as described previously. In a process-oriented evaluation, a flowchart is kept of the exact sequence and strategy the subject follows. This enables the examiner to record whether there was a great deal of trial and error, for example, or whether responses were slow but well reasoned.

9. **Object Assembly.** The subject must complete a series of four picture puzzles on this timed task, and again the examiner keeps a flowchart to monitor performance and strategies. An adaptation is to encourage the subject to name the target object as soon as it is identified and to evaluate whether he or she is proceeding with a specific target in mind or is aimlessly manipulating the pieces until they suggest something. If the subject is unable to complete the task even after the time limits have been extended, the examiner can provide additional structure in several ways. The subject who has failed to identify the figure is given this information to see if this will facilitate organization. The examiner may place critical pieces to see if the patient can utilize them constructively.

10. **Picture Arrangement.** Ten sets of pictures, each depicting a sequential social interaction, make up this timed task. Each set is presented out of order, and the subject is asked to rearrange the pieces so that they make a logical story. Standard administration specifies arrangement of the pictures from left to right, but in the case of visual field deficits, it may be preferable to lay out the cards vertically.

Although not called for in the directions, one can encourage subjects, after they have provided a solution, to describe what they think is going on. This modification can provide information about potential perceptual problems as opposed to errors of logic or sequencing. Once again, qualitative analysis of this task is often helpful; an individual with a mild sequencing problem may appreciate the "gist" of each story but misplace a single item on several. That person may achieve just as poor a score as someone who has utterly misinterpreted the situation or who has understood and sequenced each item perfectly but has done so too slowly to receive any credit.

11. **Digit Symbol.** This paper-and-pencil task evaluates the number of items in a code, which involves substituting symbols for corresponding digits, that the subject can complete within the time limits. The disadvantages of using this test to evaluate aphasic individuals has been discussed previously.

B. Wechsler Memory Scale–Revised

The original *Wechsler Memory Scale* was comprised of seven subtests, from which a unitary Memory Quotient was derived. The 1987 revision has expanded the number of subtests to include more measures of nonverbal memory and has replaced the Memory Quotient with composite indices, labeled Verbal Memory, Visual Memory, General Memory, Attention/Concentration, and Delayed Recall, in an attempt to separate factors that might be differentially affected in various types of memory disorders. Each index has a mean of 100 and standard deviation of 15, so that the indices can be readily compared with one another. In addition to data from normal individuals, the standardization included numerous clinical subgroups that have their own norms. Although norms are available for a group of patients with strokes, the sample included an equal mixture of patients with right- and left-hemisphere strokes, so that these norms are not particularly helpful in interpreting the performance of a given aphasic individual. Descriptions of the WMS-R subtests follow:

1. **Information and Orientation.** This subtest elicits information from remote memory, including biographical information and well-known general knowledge, as well as evidence of orientation to place and time. These items are

quite simple and generally are passed without difficulty by normal individuals.

2. **Mental Control.** These items tap automatized series (reciting the alphabet and counting backward from 20) as well as serial addition (counting sequentially by threes, beginning with the number 1).

3. **Figural Memory.** This multiple-choice measure involves a series of items in which the subject is exposed to a set of abstract designs. The stimulus then is removed, and the subject must identify the original designs from a larger array. Because a pointing response is all that is required of the subject, this format is amenable to testing aphasic patients with motor impairments. However, experience shows that many aphasic patients perform at least as poorly on this task as on those that require graphomotor production.

4. **Logical Memory.** The standard administration of this task calls for the examiner to read aloud two brief narrative passages. After each, the examinee is asked to recount the story in as much detail as possible. Following a 30-minute delay, the subject again is asked to recall the story. Obviously the expressive language demands of this task place the aphasic individual at a disadvantage; thus, after free recall (if indeed the individual can produce a narrative response at all) the examiner can probe by asking specific questions about the stories. Additionally, a series of multiple-choice items can be presented, both orally and in print, and the subject can indicate a response by pointing if necessary.

As noted previously, it is informative to give corrections to multiple-choice errors and to compare immediate and delayed recall multiple-choice performance. This adaptation enables one to determine, regardless of whether the initial level of recall was high or low, whether information once acquired was retained over the course of a half-hour delay or whether there was a rapid decay in new verbal learning. Not infrequently, there is actually an increase in performance on the delayed recall condition when feedback has been given after immediate recall. This pattern may be due to the fact that having one's attention specifically focused on a particular detail facilitates the ability to encode and store it. Moreover, in the presence of language-processing difficulties, the conversational pace of presentation of the story may overwhelm the patient's capacity to process and encode each bit of information before the next is presented. Parts of each story are presented in the passive voice, which can lead to confusion of agent/object relations in individuals whose comprehension of syntax is compromised.

5. **Visual Paired Associates.** In this subtest each of six colors is paired with an abstract design, and the patient subsequently must recall which color went with each design. As this is intended to be a nonverbal memory task, the names of the colors are not spoken by the examiner in an effort to discourage verbalization. It is clear, however, that many patients adopt verbal strategies; for example, one patient remembered the figure that went with the color green by telling himself that it looked like a map of Ireland. Many individuals with deficits in color naming perform poorly on this task, further suggesting that verbal encoding facilitates performance. Subjects are scored over three learning trials; additional trials (up to six) are given if the subject has not mastered the pairings. The same information is tested 30 minutes later.

6. **Verbal Paired Associates.** Here the examiner reads a list of eight word pairs, four of which are considered easy because of obvious semantic associations (e.g., "rose–flower") and four of which are difficult because they are unrelated (e.g., "cabbage–pen"). The examiner next presents the first word of each pair, and the subject must supply the one with which it had been paired. Corrections are given to erroneous responses. As with the visual paired associates, the pairs are repeated for at least three and up to six learning trials until all the word pairs are learned, but only the first three trials are scored. Delayed recall is tested after a half-hour filled delay.

7. **Visual Reproductions.** In this task four cards containing one or two simple visual designs are exposed. After each card is removed, the subject must draw the design(s) from memory. Delayed recall also is requested after some 30 minutes. One problem with this task is that an individual with motor deficits or organizational problems may have a

perfectly intact internal representation of the figures but be unable to reproduce them correctly. A copying condition may follow the delayed recall to help isolate the effects of poor drawing skill from memory. When graphomotor problems are severe, one might give a multiple-choice recognition test after the patient has attempted to draw the figure. If the examiner suspects that a severe impairment of visuospatial perception may underlie the performance deficit, he or she can try a multiple-choice matching condition, in which the patient is shown the target drawing again and must choose the design that matches it.

8. **Digit Span.** The form of this task is the same as its counterpart in WAIS-R (discussed previously).

9. **Visual Memory Span.** Here the subject is presented with a seemingly random array of nine colored squares. The examiner touches increasing numbers of them, beginning with two, with two trials at each level. After observing each sequence, the subject must touch the same squares in the same order. As with the digit span task, when maximum visual span has been reached, there is a condition in which the subject must reverse the spans, touching them in the opposite order from that demonstrated.

C. Coloured Progressive Matrices

The *Coloured Progressive Matrices* test (Raven, Court, & Raven, 1984) is a simpler version of Raven's *Standard Progressive Matrices*. Each item consists of a visual matrix from which a piece is missing; the task requires choosing from among alternatives the piece that would best complete the design. (All items are printed on a page, so that no physical manipulation of the stimulus materials is possible.) The easiest items require only simple perceptual discrimination, but the more difficult ones involve active mental manipulation of multiple stimulus dimensions as well as analogical reasoning. The task has the advantage of requiring only a pointing response, and research has shown that this test, while correlating well with verbal intelligence, is unimpaired in a high percentage of aphasic patients. Kertesz and McCabe (1975) reported that patients' scores were uncorrelated with *severity* of aphasia, but noted that Broca's, transcortical motor, conduction, and anomic aphasics generally performed as well as controls, while global, transcortical sensory, and Wernicke's aphasics obtained impaired scores when evaluated acutely.

In addition to the test's usefulness in estimating a patient's relative level of cognitive ability, some specific error types may emerge, including a serial position response bias, or a tendency to choose impulsively a piece that matches a detail of the stimulus rather than one that completes the overall pattern.

III. Boston Stimulus Board

The *Boston Stimulus Board* (Helm-Estabrooks & Kaplan, 1989) is not a formal test but rather a set of stimuli (including letters, numbers, words, colors, designs, and math problems). The accompanying task guidelines are designed to facilitate a process-oriented investigation of a variety of linguistic, memory, and conceptual abilities, particularly in patients with unreliable or limited speech output. These stimuli are presented in the form of a partitioned board, which also can serve as a pacing board for dysarthric patients. Each task is accompanied by suggestions for flexible modification according to the individual patient's needs and a discussion of the importance of specific types of errors that each task may elicit.

IV. Interpretation of Neuropsychological Test Results

In communicating results of a neuropsychological evaluation to the patient's family and to professional colleagues, try to focus on the salient features of the individual's performance. It is equally important to describe major strengths and assets as well as areas of difficulty and disability. Testing is useful insofar as the required tasks and abilities permit valid inferences about how the patient will interact with situations and stimuli in his or her everyday environment. The notion of rehabilitation is based on helping a disabled individual regain former abilities or compensate for lost skills as effectively as possible. Remediation may involve recruiting new functional systems to accomplish or to approximate the former skill. This principle has been demonstrated in aphasia therapy, for example, through the use of melodic intonation, which facilitates speech output using a singing technique (see chapter 15).

Some aphasic patients will continue to function remarkably well in nonlinguistic cognitive domains, but others will require intervention aimed at remediating deficits in attention, memory, visuospatial organization, problem-solving strategies, or vocational skills. Understanding the unique cognitive capacities an individual brings to the therapeutic situation will help point to appropriate treatment strategies. Knowing that a severely nonfluent individual has a functionally intact right hemisphere and can produce clear and recognizable drawings, for example, may suggest an avenue for communication not available to another patient with similar language problems (see chapter 13). The aphasic patient who has a marked problem in storing and retrieving new information will require a different therapeutic plan than one who has trouble learning after a single presentation but goes on to show a satisfactory learning curve across repeated trials with good retention after a delay.

The importance of a patient's motivation, awareness of cognitive problems, and skills in self-monitoring and self-correcting cannot be overemphasized. Knowledge of these variables enables the clinician to make predictions about how much structure and supervision will be required and how well the patient will be able to utilize therapy. Although the ability to generate problem-solving strategies is usually a positive sign, careful attention to the details of testing may at times identify tendencies to adopt erroneous or counterproductive strategies that can be eliminated in therapy.

As recovery progresses, the patient's abilities and needs may change substantially. In some cases, diffuse or multifocal cognitive deficits resulting from edema or poststroke metabolic changes may resolve, but in all cases language and nonlinguistic abilities alike require repeated examination to reflect an accurate and current profile of skills and assets.

The process approach to neuropsychological evaluation takes the testing situation as a microcosm of the patient's ability to interact with and adapt to the world at large. Simply drawing inferences about structural brain changes on the basis of test results is insufficient; testing should be approached as a collaborative and interactive relationship between examiner and patient. Neuropsychological testing should provide valid and useful inferences about real-life adaptive skills and how the patient can be helped to maximize his or her preserved skills in everyday settings.

References and Suggested Readings

Goodglass, H., & Kaplan, E. (1984). *The assessment of aphasia and related disorders.* Philadelphia: Lea & Febiger.

Grant, D.A., & Berg, E.A. (1981). *Wisconsin Card Sorting Test.* Odessa, FL: Psychological Assessment Resources.

Helm-Estabrooks, N., & Kaplan, E. (1989). *Boston Stimulus Board: Clinician's guide*. San Antonio, TX: Special Press.

Kaplan, E.F. (1988). A process approach to neuropsychological assessment. In T. Boll & B.K. Bryant (Eds.), *Clinical neuropsychology and brain function: Research measurement and practice* (pp. 125-167). Washington, DC: American Psychological Association.

Kaplan, E.F., Fein, D., Morris, R., & Delis, D.C. (in press). *The Wechsler Adult Intelligence Scale-Revised as a neuropsychological instrument*. San Antonio, TX: Psychological Corporation.

Kertesz, A., & McCabe, P. (1975). Intelligence and aphasia: Performance of aphasics on Raven's Coloured Progressive Matrices. *Brain & Language, 2*, 387-395.

Lezak, M. (1983). *Neuropsychological assessment*. New York: Oxford University Press.

Luria, A.R. (1973). *The working brain*. New York: Basic Books.

Raven, J.C., Court, J.H., & Raven, J. (1984). *Coloured Progressive Matrices*. London: H.K. Lewis.

Sandson, J., & Albert, M.L. (1987). Perseveration in behavioral neurology. *Neurology, 37*, 1736-1741.

Wechsler, D. (1981). *WAIS-R manual: Wechsler Adult Intelligence Scale-Revised*. San Antonio, TX: Psychological Corporation.

Wechsler, D. (1986). *WMS-R manual: Wechsler Memory Scale-Revised*. San Antonio, TX: Psychological Corporation.

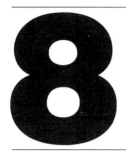

Aphasia Examination

As stated in the discussion of aphasia classification presented in chapter 3, the differential diagnosis of aphasia is based primarily on samples of discourse, auditory comprehension, repetition, and naming. Additionally, the evaluation of reading, writing, automatic speech, and singing may provide a final important dimension to the diagnostic picture. Specific techniques have been developed to evaluate each of these components of the aphasia examination, and descriptions of these follow.

I. Obtaining and Analyzing Discourse Samples

To differentiate fluent from nonfluent aphasic syndromes according to the conversational speech parameters described in chapter 3, one must obtain samples of discourse. In addition to providing information regarding the fluency/nonfluency characteristics, samples of connected speech also can be analyzed for the amount of *accurate* information conveyed, which allows one to make some judgments as to the severity of the communication deficit. The examiner can obtain connected speech samples by engaging the patient in a semistructured conversation and asking him or her to provide a narrative (expository speech) description of pictured events. Tape-recording these samples (with the patient's permission) allows for future transcription and analysis.

A. The Conversational Speech Sample

The language examination should begin with a conversation. During a relaxed conversation the patient may be able to provide important personal information or insight into the problem at hand. Additionally, the patient's self-formulated responses tell the examiner about the nature of the aphasia. Begin the conversation in a natural way with social exchanges and short-answer questions of biographical facts; progress to open-ended questions that elicit longer speech samples. In addition to personally relevant questions, ask at least one question relating to a well-known, highly emotional, historical event (for example, in the *Aphasia Diagnostic Profiles* [Helm-Estabrooks, 1991], questions are asked about the assassination of President Kennedy or the assassination of John Lennon, depending on the age of the patient). Some patients, of course, will give short, incomplete answers, so that the examiner must probe for more information in an attempt to elicit longer runs of speech. Avoid the use of yes/no and multiple-choice questions except with the most impaired patients.

Although tape-recording is recommended for later analysis of the speech parameters, the experienced clinician can rate these parameters "on-line" if taping is not possible. In either case, the conversational speech sample can be used to distinguish fluent from nonfluent cortical aphasia syndromes and to "flag" those patients who show the fluent and nonfluent features suggestive of subcortical aphasia.

1. Conversation interview

The following example provides a workable structure for collecting the conversational sample:

a. "I'm (Dr., Mrs., Mr., Ms.) (Full Name). What is *your* full name?

b. "And your full address?"

c. "Well, it's nice to meet you. How are you feeling today?"

d. "What *happened* to you?"

e. "What is your biggest problem now?"

f. "Tell me about your family." (If probes are needed, try to keep them as open-ended as possible; e.g., "Do you have children? Tell me about them.")

g. "What did you do for a living? Tell me about your job."

h. "Do you remember President Kennedy? What happened to him?" (Depending on the completeness of the patient's answer, one can probe for specific information on this item; e.g., "When was that?" "Where did that happen?" "Who shot him?" "What happened to Oswald?" "Who shot him" "Who became the next president?")

The following conversational responses were obtained from patients with fluent, nonfluent, and subcortical aphasia. Of course, in order to judge such important speech features as melodic line and articulatory agility, these samples must be heard; however, other features such as grammatical form, phrase length, word finding, and paraphasias can be judged from the written transcript.

2. **Elicited speech samples**

   a. **Probe: "What happened to you?"**

   (Fluent Aphasia) "On Sunday I get up. I feel find, but on Monday . . . I have as many to . . . . A man who believes to me and I am talking to him about what I am doing and this man is a new man and he says . . . 'Al . . . you're doing . . . . I have your stuff on reddin' in ere . . . but you cannot talk to me today. I cannot take your . . . I do not know what you're saying to me well. I want you to do with one of the girls to your doctor and go him on Monday and the girl takes me in her car to doctors.'"

   Although this patient sometimes cut his sentences short ("I have as many to ——"), he produced sentences up to 28 words long in this small sample. These sentences contained a range of grammatical forms, but sometimes words were misused (**paragrammatism**) as in "believes *to* me." There were relatively few content words and frequent substitutions of vague terms ("a man," "stuff"), so that the listener has only a sense of what happened. This patient also performed poorly on auditory comprehension and repetition tests. The diagnosis was Wernicke's aphasia.

   (Nonfluent Aphasia) "I had . . . a stroke. We'd just . . . finished . . . ah . . . patrol. And the . . . ah . . . . We had . . . debris. I didn't go . . . because . . . I was . . . well . . . I had a stroke . . . in the middle . . . of the night. And bring me . . . to the hospital. Then go here . . . to get . . . therapy."

   In this sample, the patient produces no more than three words in any breath group. Grammatical form, while not severely limited, is compromised. There is one apparent literal **paraphasia** (*debris* for *debriefing*). Content words, however, convey more information than in the preceding sample of fluent aphasia. Further testing showed that auditory comprehension was relatively preserved while repetition was limited to single words and short, high frequency phrases. The diagnosis was Broca's aphasia.

b.   **Probe: "What is your major problem now?"**

(Fluent Aphasia) "Putting my words together. I can't seem to get 'em together. I can't seem to get 'em together, that's what it is. The words that don't appear in front of 'em, you know. Like the words are coming . . . supposed to come out . . . and I have to think sometimes what word am I supposed to be using here and . . . like little funny things . . . and they, they'll come out automatically most of the time and other times, the same word . . . I say 'Well what do I use for that word?' 'Is it "glass"?' I'll be thinking."

The major problem experienced by this patient was word finding, as he himself described. Instead of specific words, he used vague terms such as "little funny things." Beyond this, he demonstrated no paraphasias. Formal testing showed that auditory comprehension and repetition were essentially spared, consistent with a diagnosis of anomic aphasia.

(Mixed Aphasia) "My speech and other stuff too. My hand is not good. The leg is not good. The brain I think is good but not good enough. And brain and mouth workin' together is good. I know it is this way but I cannot do it myself in my head."

As in the preceding sample of fluent anomic aphasia, this patient had a primary difficulty in word finding, although he had somewhat better access to substantive words. Within the sample, phrase length varied from 5 to 15 words. Similarly, grammatical form varied greatly. In such a case, the examiner has difficulty in judging whether this is fluent or nonfluent speech. When features of both fluent and nonfluent speech present, this often is an indication that the diagnosis is subcortical aphasia. The finding that auditory comprehension was virtually intact in this patient and that repetition was good for high frequency sentences further suggested a subcortical form of aphasia, which subsequently was confirmed by CT scan.

3. **With exercises in the manner just illustrated, analyze the following samples and make a diagnostic judgment:**

    a. **Probe: "What did you do for a living?"**

    (Sample 1) "A nurse where I'm a nurse but I cown in Maine now. I can say the part but the rest I can't say." (Examiner: "While in the service?") "Well we want to . . . went down . . . in there. Instead of me put in nursing they stuck me where they cook and anything. That's for . . . no, when I went. I started in a place . . . have a place where they . . . oh, I know what it is, but I can't. It's a place we had there . . . we had uh . . . high, you know, off . . . oh how do you say it? Well, anyway, the men play . . . they lived and had a plane . . . and then they lived on the case they lived there . . . their cars were there where they lived with the cars or automobiles. Oh, I'm all mixed up."

    Repetition and auditory comprehension in this case were moderately impaired.

    (Sample 2) "Ma-son." (Examiner: "What kind?") "Outdoors. Bwicks."

    Auditory comprehension was relatively good while repetition was poor.

    (Sample 3) "Cabbie . . . cab driver . . . yes . . . for about seven years. (Examiner: "What else?") "Ah-tel work . . . worked with hotels . . . bell captain mainly . . . and then sales." (Examiner: "What kind?") "Ma-ma-major appliances."

    Both auditory comprehension and repetition were relatively spared in this case.

    (The diagnoses for these samples are found at the end of this chapter.)

B. The Expository Speech Sample

In addition to the sample of speech elicited within the context of a conversation, an expository description of a pictured scene

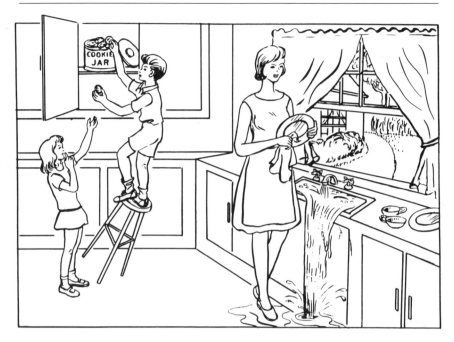

FIG. 8.1. "Cookie Theft" (From *Boston Diagnostic Aphasia Examination* by Harold Goodglass and Edith Kaplan. Copyright 1983 by Lea & Febiger. Reprinted by permission.)

should be obtained. There are many reasons for presenting an expository speech task, among them that (a) the demands on memory are reduced, (b) the patient must retrieve specific words, (c) the picture organizes the narrative, (d) the examiner knows the precise targets (which is not true of conversational attempts), and (e) the picture description can be used to compare patients to each other and to themselves at different time intervals.

The examples that follow here are narrative descriptions of the "Cookie Theft" picture (Fig. 8.1) from the *Boston Diagnostic Aphasia Examination* (Goodglass & Kaplan, 1984). However, any picture in which there are people and objects engaged in activities and accidents can be used as effectively (e.g., a fruit-picking scene in which one man is falling from a ladder and another is being chased by a dog while a third is filling his sack).

If the examiner creates a new picture, norms must be obtained by recording descriptions given by nonaphasic persons matched to the examiner's typical aphasic population in terms of sex, age, race, handedness, occupation, and education. This will allow, by performing a set of analyses (such as those described in chapter 11), the creation of a yardstick against which to measure the performance of aphasic patients.

1. Sample descriptions of "Cookie Theft" picture

(Anomic Aphasia) "I see someone almost fallin' down. And this . . . this person up here . . . she . . . . This is about to fall down and somebody's tryin' to get something out here. . . . The food or something up on top there . . . takin' something out. And there's someone losing here to somebody . . . runnin' on the floor. That's not right! Somebody could get hurt. It's runnin' out." (Examiner: "What?") "The water is running' out on the floor." (Examiner: "And here?") "This person's tryin' to get whatever they're tryin' to get. They're about to fall down here. And this girl here is trying to give something to here that's up here. It could have been . . . she could have been here. She looks like she's goin' to be cleanin' up the place. She's not doin' a good job with it."

This description was produced with good intonation and normal articulation. Average, occasional phrase length exceeds seven words, although some sentences are cut short because of word-finding problems. In addition, grammatical form is normal, suggesting a form of fluent aphasia. There are no obvious paraphasias, but the sample is relatively empty of substantive words, so that only six accurate pieces of information about the picture are conveyed. When this number is divided into the total number of words produced (126), one can see that the patient uses an average of 21 words to express each bit of information. This is far greater than the normal average of about four words per bit of information. One can conclude then that this fluent aphasic patient has notable word-finding difficulty, which, in the absence of paraphasias, indicates anomic aphasia.

(Transcortical Motor Aphasia) "Cookie jar. Falling. Surprise." (Examiner: "Over here?") "Water running to waste." (Examiner: "Give me a full sentence.") "The boy is falling." (Examiner: "Anything else?") "Surprise." (Examiner: "Give me a full sentence.") "Surprise is . . . ."

This patient's description was produced with good articulation, but the short phrase length interrupted the melodic line. The longest statements consisted of only four words but formed simple sentences. These sentences occurred only after a clinician's probe. There are no paraphasias, and the patient manages to produce five bits of accurate information in only 17 words for an average of 3.4 words per content unit (below the average of 4 words per content unit). Limited speech output with short phrase length, simple grammatical form, and relatively good word finding in the absence of paraphasia suggests transcortical motor aphasia. Another hallmark of this syndrome is inertia of speech production, so that the clinician must probe constantly for more output. The diagnosis is confirmed if repetition and auditory comprehension skills are relatively spared.

II. Evaluating Auditory Comprehension Skills

A. Basic Concepts in Testing

Any test of auditory comprehension assumes that the patient has intact output pathways; that is, a means of reliably demonstrating an understanding of the spoken word. It is known, however, that conditions such as severe apraxia may interfere with simple pointing responses and the ability to indicate "yes" or "no." Of course, a diagnosis of impaired auditory comprehension also assumes that the patient has the peripheral hearing skills necessary for discriminating spoken words. Ideally, an audiological evaluation precedes the auditory comprehension exam, so that hearing deficits are not confounding the results.

Other problems that are extrinsic to auditory comprehension skills but that can interfere with performance may be visual or visuospatial in nature. Some aphasic patients have a right homonomous hemianopia that prevents them from seeing items located to the right side of their midline. More aphasic patients than it is generally appreciated may manifest inattention to the right side of space. Others may have difficulty in visually discriminating or scanning pictured stimuli to make correct choices. Finally, when stimuli exceed a single word in length, auditory-verbal memory may interfere with performance. Thus, a well-designed comprehension exam must make every effort to circumvent deficits such as apraxia, hearing loss, and visuospatial impairment that, although extrinsic to auditory comprehension, may interfere with accurate assessment. Only then can a clinician make judgments as to the relative preservation or impairment of this language modality.

In the differential diagnosis of aphasia, we speak of **relative impairment** and **relative preservation** of various aspects of language. In the case of auditory comprehension, it is possible that no aphasic patient experiences a total loss of the ability to understand auditory messages. Similarly, few aphasic patients have total preservation of auditory comprehension. To test this contention, however, one would have to design an examination that could capture small islands of preserved ability in severely impaired patients and at the same time challenge those with mild impairment. An effective auditory comprehension test, therefore, is comprised of a variety of tasks, including single-word, sentence, and paragraph discrimination, and single and multistep commands. Within each of these tasks, certain types of material may be relatively easier or harder for a particular patient. To assess this variability of performance from category to category, a thorough exam will include material representing a range of semantic and syntactic classes as well as controlling such variables as emotionality, personal relevance, and frequency of occurrence.

Clinical and research experience with aphasic patients shows that, as a group, they respond better to questions regarding their personal life (e.g., "Are you married?") than to more neutral questions of fact (e.g., "Is it sunny?"). Natural and/or frequently occurring commands (e.g., "Pull up your chair") are followed more accurately than unlikely commands (e.g., "Slap the book"). Frequency of occurrence is a powerful variable (e.g., *chair* vs. *hassock*), but emotionality may outweigh frequency (e.g., *gun* vs. *spoon*). These same factors are relevant to comprehension of paragraphs, so that stories about daily events (either humorous or tragic) may be understood better than narratives relating impersonal facts. Of course, length and grammatical complexity play a powerful role in the comprehension of commands, sentences, and paragraphs.

Remember: Aphasic patients may have peripheral hearing losses involving speech frequencies. If possible, an audiological evaluation is obtained early. But in any case, the examiner should speak clearly, use good volume, and maintain eye contact with the patient as each stimulus is presented.

In addition, the effective auditory comprehension exam begins with items having high probability of eliciting a correct response and proceeds to ones that present a greater challenge to aphasic patients.

B. Testing Comprehension of Commands

Intuitively one might assume that single words are easier for aphasic patients to understand than longer utterances. However, this is not necessarily the case. Some severely aphasic patients may perform poorly when asked to point to pictures in response to spoken single words and yet show good comprehension of sentence-length commands given within a natural context (e.g., "Pull your chair a little closer"). In addition, these patients may perform so-called axial or whole body commands (e.g., "Stand like a boxer") with relative ease. An analysis of responses made by a group of 45 globally aphasic patients given the *Boston Assessment of Severe Aphasia* (Helm-Estabrooks, Ramsberger, Morgan, & Nicholas, 1989) showed that over 90% responded correctly to the command "Close your eyes." Despite such observations, many clinicians continue to judge a patient's ability to understand spoken commands solely on the basis of unlikely instructions such as "Place the yellow pencil under the blue book." Granted, this latter type of command might be valuable in assessing subtler comprehension deficits in patients with mild impairments, but their exclusive use may yield an inaccurate picture of comprehension in more severely involved patients.

Begin an auditory comprehension exam with commands rather than with a test of single-word discrimination, as commands can be delivered naturally at the beginning of the exam. For example, after obtaining the samples of connected speech, the examiner can give the following instructions in a casual tone without gesturing:

1. "Now move your chair a little closer."

2. "Could you sit up straighter?"

3. "Please close your eyes." (If the patient does not reopen them, so instruct him or her.)

4. "Okay, now look around the room."

5. "Where are the lights?"

6. "And where is the door?"

7. "Point to the source of illumination."

8. "Show me the entry way to this room."

Interestingly, clinical experience has shown patients unable to point to the lights or door carry out commands such as "Turn off the lights" or "Shut the door." Patients who cannot point to their eyeglasses may respond to "Take off your glasses" with no hesitation. These observations underscore the fact that most patients do better with commands in natural contexts.

The single-step (requiring only one action) commands listed above may present little challenge to the less impaired patient. For this reason, a variety of objects can be placed before the patient and longer, multistep commands offered (e.g., "Fold the dollar in half and place it in the envelope along with the quarter"). With these longer, more complex commands, the examiner notes the pieces or parts of the command that are processed correctly. In the preceding command, for example, the patient might put the dollar in the envelope without folding it in half and ignore the quarter. In keeping with the process approach, note any aberrant behavior such as perseveration.

Remember: Few (if any) aphasic patients totally lack the ability to process information presented auditorily. On the other hand, few (if any) aphasic patients have totally intact auditory comprehension. A good exam will tease out both intact abilities in severely impaired patients and impaired abilities in mildly impaired patients.

Furthermore, in all testing of auditory comprehension, the process approach dictates that the examiner note exactly what the patient did in response to the stimulus.

C. Testing Comprehension of Single Words

Although a seemingly artificial task, it is important to determine the extent to which aphasic patients can process single words. One reason for testing single-word comprehension is that many patients show semantic category differences in word recognition (e.g., color names vs. object names). Furthermore, differences in ability to process certain semantic categories may have diagnostic value. Some patients with Wernicke's aphasia, for example, may show relative difficulty in understanding the names of letters and body parts.

Another reason for testing single-word comprehension is that it is diagnostically important to observe whether patients spontaneously and correctly repeat the word offered to them and yet fail to identify the correct item. This suggests one of two phenomena: word/meaning alienation or visuoperceptual problems. In the first instance, although the patient can repeat the item and therefore has "heard" the word, the particular combination of sounds no longer carries meaning. This phenomenon may be indicative of transcortical sensory aphasia, where patients easily repeat even long sentences without comprehension. In the second instance, a patient may understand the meaning of the word but choose incorrectly because he or she cannot visually discriminate or decode the stimuli. When presented with material that does not require visual processing (e.g., listening to paragraphs and answering related questions), however, such a patient may show good comprehension.

1. **Choosing and presenting single-word stimuli.** Some aphasic patients recognize the names of semantic categories (e.g., "colors," "numbers," "flowers," "animals") and yet fail to recognize the names of specific items within these categories (e.g., "red," "lion"). The single-word comprehension exam, therefore, may begin by presenting items in semantic groups and asking the patient to point to, for example, "the letters."

   To overcome or minimize visual or visuospatial problems, present the choices (either semantic groups of items or single items) in a vertical array, with line drawings on a black background. Shading of items may lend further visual salience. To overcome or minimize the effect of peripheral hearing problems, the patient should look directly at the examiner when the verbal stimuli are offered.

In choosing items for a test of single-word comprehension, consider the following factors that may influence aphasic performance:

Number of syllables

Word frequency

Emotionality

Semantic category

Phonemic similarity

These factors will influence both comprehension of the names of semantic categories and the items within these categories. It is recommended that the clinician test auditory comprehension of single words within the semantic categories of objects, actions, letters, numbers, and colors.

Finally, it should be noted that many aphasic patients (including those with so-called "global aphasia") may show relative strength in understanding geographic place names; thus, use an outline map of the patient's homeland to test this ability.

2. **Recording and analyzing responses.** In keeping with the process approach, the examiner should record the patient's exact response to each verbal stimulus. Further, it is important to note the order in which the stimuli were presented; this allows for an analysis of perseveration (repeated selection of an item in response to a new stimulus word). Delays over 5 seconds should be noted as well as self-corrections.

Important questions to ask are the following:

a. Does the patient recognize and distinguish the names of semantic categories, for example "letters" from "colors"?

b. Does the patient respond correctly but slowly?

c. Does the patient perseverate on choices?

   d. Does the patient show awareness of difficulty?

   e. Does the patient display particular strengths for some semantic categories and particular weaknesses for others?

D. Testing Comprehension of Sentences and Paragraphs

It is important to assess the patient's understanding of spoken sentences and paragraphs regardless of performance on other auditory comprehension tasks. There are several reasons for this, including the possibility that connected speech may reflect more closely the kinds of material one is expected to understand in everyday situations. People rarely speak in single, isolated words, but instead communicate through connected discourse. If aphasic patients are to function at even a moderately successful level in society, they must demonstrate the ability to understand some discourse. It may be, in fact, that connected speech samples are easier to understand than single words because they are redundant and carry important suprasegmental (e.g., prosody and stress) and contextual information.

In constructing or choosing paragraphs, the clinician should be aware of certain factors that may influence or bias performance. For example, one should avoid material that conveys information for which some patients, but not others, may have prior knowledge (e.g., a paragraph on fly fishing). Unique stories are best, and those with some degree of emotionality or humor may enhance performance. Paragraphs should have both stated and unstated, or inferred, main ideas and details, as in the examples that follow. Once again, "yes/no" questions are paired to minimize the chance effect. It is important to pose the questions in a way so as not to suggest a yes or no response to the patient. Finally, the clinician should try to rule out impaired memory as the cause of poor performance.

In the following paragraph, taken from Helm-Estabrooks, Gress, and Sperry (in press), the questions are constructed to probe for understanding of both the stated and inferred main ideas and details:

My cousin was lost in the mountains when a blinding snowstorm hit while she was hiking. Her food supplies ran out in two days. Melted snow kept her alive until she was found five days later. She was rescued when a helicopter spotted her red scarf.

1. **Stated main idea:**

   a. Was my cousin hiking in the mountains when she got lost?

   b. Was my cousin skiing in the mountains when she got lost?

2. **Stated detail:**

   a. Did she eat red berries to stay alive?

   b. Did she eat melted snow to stay alive?

3. **Inferred main idea:**

   a. Was my cousin lost because she was blind?

   b. Was my cousin lost because of a snowstorm?

4. **Inferred detail:**

   a. Did a helicopter find her?

   b. Did hunters find her?

III. Evaluating Repetition Skills

A. Basic Concepts in Testing

Always explore aphasic patients' repetition skills because the ability to repeat can be used for distinguishing syndromes within the fluent and nonfluent categories (e.g., conduction aphasia vs. anomic aphasia, Broca's aphasia vs. transcortical motor aphasia). The evaluation of repetition, in fact, is a crucial part of any aphasia exam.

Tests of repetition skills presuppose that the patient has the peripheral hearing, attention, and memory skills necessary for performing this task. If, for example, a patient produces the word *tea* in response to the word *key,* one should rule out hearing as a source of the error. Once adequacy of peripheral hearing has been established, one is ready to evaluate repetition skills, beginning with single words.

B. Single-Word Repetition

Many of the same parameters that influence performance on other language tasks will affect repetition performance: word frequency, semantic category, emotionality, and phonemic complexity, length, and grammatical form.

In keeping with the process approach, one should transcribe and analyze all responses for articulatory errors; literal, verbal, or neologistic paraphasias; and augmentation and paraphrasing. The nature of the material that elicits both the best and poorest performances also is noted (a tape recorder will facilitate this process). Typically, begin with repeating single-syllable words that start with easily visualized, voiced consonants (e.g., *bed*). Blends and multisyllable words are introduced later (e.g., *cloudy*). Object names are contrasted with verbs, numbers, letters, and functor words, because some patients show strengths or weaknesses among these categories. Other patients may find only "tongue twisters" difficult (e.g., *happy hippopotamus*), while those with severely restricted speech may only repeat their own stereotypic expressions (e.g., "oh boy").

C. Repetition of Sentences

The exam for sentence-length repetition skills begins with short, frequently occurring stimuli, such as "Sit down." These are contrasted with short, infrequently occurring sentences, such as "Tap the keg." These paired sentences can become gradually longer and grammatically more complex (e.g., "When you go out, buy a newspaper" vs. "When you scuba dive, wear a rubber suit"). The following items capture some of the variables important to a simple test of repetition:

1. Bed

2. Five

3. Wash

4. D

5. Cloudy

6. Eighty-seven

7. Struggling

8. A

9. I love you.

10. She is here.

11. Babies cry.

12. Lobsters molt.

13. If he comes, I will go.

14. After you turn the knob, push the button.

15. She sold six silk sheets.

IV. Evaluating Naming Skills

A. Basic Concepts in Testing

As stated previously, virtually all aphasic patients have difficulty in naming, although the underlying reasons for this
difficulty vary according to aphasia type. Even within an individual patient, the reason for misnaming may depend on the
nature of the task. In addition, the performance of the aphasic
patient will be influenced by physical states such as stress and
fatigue. When testing naming skills in aphasia patients, one
must make every effort to control factors that, although extrinsic to the basic task, may influence naming performance. Some
of these are confusion, attention, auditory comprehension deficits, fatigue, and visuospatial problems.

First, of course, the clinician should assure that the patient
understands the task, that he or she knows what is expected.
For example, one method of testing naming is that of **responsive naming**, where the patient is asked a question designed to
elicit a specific response (i.e., "What do you use to sweep the
floor?"). If the patient has auditory comprehension deficits, he
or she may respond incorrectly or not at all to such a question.
As a rule of thumb, therefore, the clinician might avoid the use
of responsive naming when auditory comprehension is in
serious question; however, if one decides to *attempt* this type of
naming with a patient having frank auditory comprehension
deficits and an incorrect response is forthcoming, a judgment
must be made (based on the nature of the error) as to whether
the error represents aphasic misnaming or lack of understanding. This judgment does not always come easily. In the case of
the question "What do you use to sweep the floor?", an answer
of "A mop" may represent a verbal/semantic paraphasia or a
failure to decode the word *sweep*. An answer of "Brown" is
unlikely to represent an aphasic misnaming error; it suggests
instead an auditory comprehension problem because it is not
within semantic category. An answer like "A kroom," on the

other hand, suggests that the question was understood but that it elicited a literal (phonemic) paraphasia.

As when testing single-word auditory comprehension, visuospatial problems can influence naming performance. When testing naming, the clinician should be certain that the patient clearly discerns the item stimulus picture. Chapter 10 offers the example of a patient who calls a harmonica "a double-decker bus." This represents a visuoperceptual naming error suggestive of right-hemisphere disease because the patient obviously attended to the details (the two rows of air holes were interpreted as windows) but failed to process the outer configuration. Left-hemisphere damage also may result in impaired visual processing, but in these cases there may be a failure to attend to crucial details. Thus, with presentation of pictures for confrontation naming, the stimuli should be clearly drawn and oriented more to visual contour than to detail. Before leaving the important point of visual discrimination, we should consider the rare syndrome of **visual agnosia**, in which the patient fails to recognize the meaning of items perceived through the visual modality. If this syndrome is suspected, several alternative approaches to naming should be taken, including presentation of real items through other modalities such as tactile or olfactory exploration. Responsive naming also may help in making this differential diagnosis.

B. Confrontation Naming

Perhaps the most frequently used task with aphasic persons is that of confrontation naming; that is, showing the patient an object or picture and asking "What is this?" Patients with severe forms of aphasia may have difficulty producing correct names for common objects such as *shoe,* while patients with mild aphasia may have difficulty only with uncommon objects, such as *abacus.* Regional factors of course will influence stimulus choices: Obviously an item like *abacus* may be easier for someone from Beijing than from Boston. The examiner must consider also whether a particular word was ever a part of the patient's vocabulary before attributing the naming problems to aphasia. In addition to word frequency, factors that will influence naming performance include the semantic category the item represents, the length and phonemic complexity of the word, and possibly the emotional value it has for the individual. Taking these factors into consideration, one can see that real objects may have limited use in a naming task. For this reason, the use of pictures allows the clinician to explore naming skills more fully.

As stated previously, a complete confrontation naming test includes high- and low-frequency items representing the following semantic categories: objects, actions, letters, numbers, colors, and body parts. If line drawings are used, the items should clearly depict the target without a reliance on small details. Shaded drawings may overcome figure/ground problems and add visual saliency to the item. The process approach dictates recording the patient's exact response to the naming task. The examiner also should record the order in which he or she presents the items so that perseverative responses can be noted.

Fig. 8.2 illustrates, via a scored subtest form, a patient's responses elicited on the Confrontation Naming subtest of the *Boston Diagnostic Aphasia Examination*. Note first that the clinician did not merely place checkmarks beside the items but instead recorded the patient's actual responses, which provide important diagnostic information beyond the raw score. In addition, her notation that the patient was "slow to get into set" raises at least two possibilities: (a) the patient has severe auditory comprehension problems so that he does not understand the verbal instructions to name the items, or (b) the patient is confused, which may represent bilateral disease or dysfunction. In any case, the clinician established set by providing a sentence completion cue, "You sit in a _____," which elicited the correct answer (for which the patient receives no credit, of course).

After saying "I don't know" (IDK) to the first two items (*chair* and *key*), the patient correctly and immediately identified *glove*. Next he said "leaf" for *feather,* which suggests visuoperceptual problems. From *hammock* he focused on the "tree," but when refocused he correctly named the item. *Cactus* was named correctly after a delay. When presented with the first item in the next section, the patient immediately identified it correctly as the letter *H*. All other responses to letters were "I don't know" except for the third response, a recurrent perseveration of the word *tree*. In all the patient earned 3 points for naming one letter in this section, as opposed to the 7 points achieved for objects.

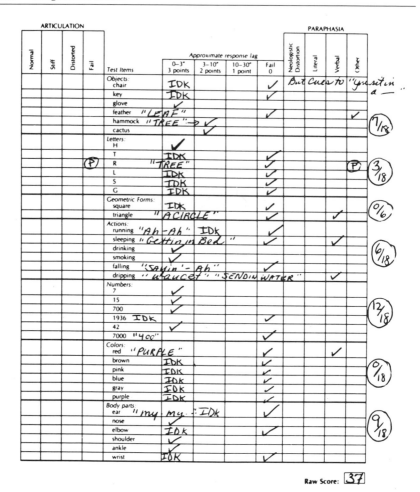

FIG. 8.2. Confrontation Naming subtest responses (From *Boston Diagnostic Aphasia Examination* by Harold Goodglass and Edith Kaplan. Copyright 1984 by Lea & Febiger. Reprinted by permission.)

Although the patient earned no points in the next section (naming geometic forms), one can see from the response "A circle" that he was in the correct semantic set. Next, in naming actions, the patient earned full credit for two items. For two others he provided no information (i.e., "I don't know" for *running;* "Sayin' ah" for *falling),* and for the remaining two he gave approximate, but related, responses (i.e., "Gettin' in bed" for *sleeping;* "Sendin' water" for *dripping).* In the substantive responses one can see a tendency to augment, not to limit the answer to the progressive verb.

Despite his poor performance in naming actions, this patient went on to name the first three numbers in the next section correctly and immediately. He then said "I don't know" for *1936* but had no trouble with *42*. Unfortunately, the "4" contaminated his next response and he produced a perseverative "400" for *7000*. In all the patient earned 12/18 points for numbers, his strongest semantic category. Color naming, on the other hand, became his weakest category; after saying "purple" for *red*, he gave up. He finished the test with an "all or none" performance on body parts naming; three were named immediately and three were "I don't know."

In all, this patient earned 37/114 points on this test of visual confrontation naming. Reporting only the overall score, however, would overlook the fact that he performed very poorly with letters and colors and relatively well with numbers, with object, action, and body part naming falling somewhere in between. In order to treat naming in this patient, one would use this hierarchy of difficulty, beginning with the patient's strongest category. But beyond his categorical raw scores, some of this patient's behavior (difficulty establishing set, visuoperceptual problems) suggest that he should be examined further for signs of bilateral involvement. Although this may be accomplished by a CT scan, the absence of a right-hemisphere lesion on the X ray does not preclude right-hemisphere disease. Instead, a thorough neuropsychological assessment might provide important additional evidence of right-hemisphere involvement.

C. Responsive Naming

Responsive naming refers to a task wherein the patient provides a substantive word in response to a contextually related question (e.g., "What color is snow?"). If the question is understood, it will provide semantic associations that will facilitate word retrieval. In the preceding example, snow is strongly related to the word *white,* as in "Snow White." This task, therefore, will be somewhat easier than if the clinician were simply to point to his or her lab coat and ask "What color is this?" Similarly, one can test retrieval of other word categories such as action words (e.g., "What do you do with scissors?") and nouns (e.g., "What do you use to write on the blackboard?"). If the patient has sufficient auditory comprehension for this task, then the results can be compared with those elicited by a confrontation naming task.

D. Categorical Naming

Free recall of items within a specific semantic category such as animals is the most difficult form of naming for aphasic patients. Although the average, nonaphasic individual can produce in excess of 20 animal names in 1 minute of free recall, even mildly aphasic patients may have difficulty in achieving this level of performance. Furthermore, free recall of animal names is a sensitive test of early-stage dementia, so it has important diagnostic implications for patients who may perform within normal limits on confrontation naming tests. For severely aphasic patients, category naming may be simply too difficult and therefore not informative.

Typically one can begin the category naming task by establishing set in the following way: "I want to see how many animals you can name. They can be zoo animals, jungle animals, farm animals, animals that live in the ocean, even animals you'd find around the house. For example, you can start with *dog.*" The most predictable response to this is "cat" and then perhaps "mouse." After that, most normals switch to another group with highly familiar names such as "cow" and "horse." A typical strategy is to cluster animals into categories such as those listed in the cue above. Within these categories normals may produce subcategories such as "The Big Cats" (e.g., lion, tiger, panther, cheetah) or simply "Big African Animals" (e.g., elephant, rhino, hippo). Some aphasic patients, however, do not "cluster" in this manner but instead produce scattered responses such as "pig . . . monkey . . . fish." Sometimes the patient will lose set, as in one (an owner of an Italian restaurant) who said "cow, horse, chicken, veal, pork, meatballs." This loss of set may be indicative of bilateral disease. In this case the clinician reestablished set by saying "Have you ever been to the zoo? What animals did you see there?"

Although it is suggested that the examiner credit only the best 1-minute performance, he or she can allow the patient up to 3 minutes to produce responses. Other semantic categories that might be tested in a similar way are makes of automobiles, fruits and vegetables, and articles of clothing.

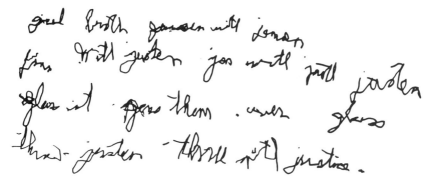

FIG. 8.3. Narrative writing: subcortical aphasia

V. Evaluating Writing Skills

A. Basic Concepts in Testing

Writing relies upon linguistic, motoric, praxic, visuospatial, and kinesthetic processes. Consequently, agraphia may be characterized by errors in spelling, syntax, and semantics, or by poor construction of the physical features of the written word. In testing the aphasic patient's writing ability, it is important to assess the influence of all of these processes on written output.

B. Graphomotor Skills Versus Linguistic Writing Skills

The graphomotor aspects of writing refer to the formation and execution of letters and symbols. Assessment of graphomotor skills should be both quantitative and qualitative. Quantitatively one notes whether the left or right hand is used, whether the patient produces printed letters or script, and whether he or she produces both upper- and lowercase letters. Within these parameters the clinician must judge legibility qualitatively, allowing, where relevant, for use of the nondominant or weakened dominant hand.

In Fig. 8.3, a patient with subcortical aphasia has used script in his attempt to write a description of the "Cookie Theft" picture. He wrote with his nondominant left hand because of right-sided paralysis. (The use of script instead of printing in this case is somewhat unusual, in that many right-handed

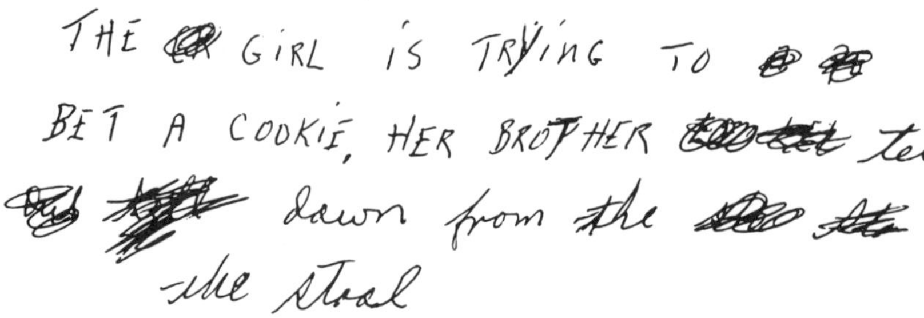

FIG. 8.4. Narrative writing: conduction aphasia

patients and normals resort to printing when forced to use their left hand.) All the letters are lowercase except for one; thus, the first thing to note is that this patient spontaneously wrote in lowercase script with his nondominant left hand. Now, looking at the **quality** of the writing (setting content aside), it is somewhat less precise than might be expected from someone using the nondominant hand. This patient, then, has graphomotor problems that could interfere with interpretation of content. In fact, only a few words are relatively legible (e.g., *them, glass*), while a few others can be guessed (e.g., *girl, broth, justice*). This writing sample provides little information to a reader unfamiliar with the picture.

In contrast, the writing sample presented in Fig. 8.4 (again describing "Cookie Theft") was obtained from a patient with conduction aphasia, who wrote with a weak right hand. He began by printing and then tried script. His printing is all uppercase, whereas the script is lowercase. The patient's formation of letters, however, is what might be expected from someone writing with a weak dominant hand, so that he does not display notable graphomotor problems. Analysis of **content** indicates that this man has word-finding and spelling problems (e.g., he begins to write *girl* as "CR-," and then writes "tell" for *fell*). In many ways this written sample reflects the patient's speech output, which is grammatically correct with literal/ phonemic paraphasias. In fact, within the context of the sentences, it is quite easy to guess what this patient meant to write. In this case, then, the spelling errors are not as detrimental to meaning as they might be if they occurred as isolated words (as in Fig. 8.5).

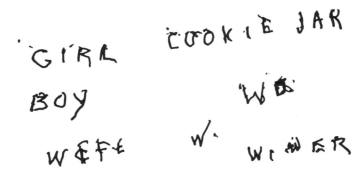

FIG. 8.5. Narrative writing: Broca's aphasia

In Fig. 8.5, a patient with severe nonfluent aphasia has printed six words, four of which convey correct information ("girl," "cookie jar," "boy"). Because the words *cookie jar* appear in the picture, he self-formulated only two correct words. Knowing the picture, one might guess that this patient also tried to write *wife* and possibly *water,* but unlike the patient with conduction aphasia, he does not provide the proper context for a naive reader to interpret these errors.

Note: When evaluating writing skills in aphasic patients, use unlined, 8½″ × 11″ paper placed lengthwise and a medium-point, black felt-tip pen (so the patient cannot erase evidence of errors). Offer a new piece of paper for each writing task (e.g., narrative writing or automatic series) to minimize perseveration or set difficulties. If the patient has right-sided hemiplegia, secure the paper lengthwise in a clipboard with the clip to the right.

For patients who are unable to write, explore spelling skills by asking them to select and arrange anagrams or use the typewriter.

C. Automatic Writing Versus Propositional Writing

There are a few writing tasks that most adults perform automatically. Among these are writing one's own name, counting consecutive numbers, and writing the alphabet, all of which are tasks learned during early school years. Similarly, words with regular spellings, learned at a young age (e.g., *cat, baby*), are produced with more ease than irregularly spelled words (e.g., *gnu* or *sphinx*) that are acquired later, if at all. With this in mind, one can begin a writing test by asking patients to write their own name. (Interestingly, clinical experience reveals some patients who have more difficulty signing their name on a blank sheet of paper than on the dotted line of a form, suggesting that context can affect performance in writing as in other tasks.) But the ability to write one's name, because of its automatic, overlearned nature, should never, by itself, be taken as evidence of intact writing skills.

D. Confrontation Writing Versus Writing to Dictation

In testing aphasic patients, it is useful to compare written communication with spoken communication. To this end, the clinician might ask a patient to write the names of pictured items (such as those listed previously in the confrontation naming section). Some patients perform better when asked to write words to dictation than when they must retrieve the words themselves. In these cases, a comparison of the two tasks allows the examiner to distinguish spelling problems from word-finding problems. In assessing spelling to dictation, however, one must be certain that the patient has the auditory skills necessary for understanding the stimuli.

Some of the items used for testing repetition (see preceding section) can be used to test writing to dictation, beginning with letters and single-syllable words and progressing to sentences. The clinician may want to add some words with irregular spelling such as *photograph* or *sugar* to probe for phonetic spelling errors (e.g., "fotograf" or "shooger"). Phonetic misspelling may be indicative of a developmental spelling problem or a low level of education, but it also occurs in some forms of aphasia.

E. Narrative Writing

A test of writing skills should assess both the ability to produce words for single items and the ability to narrate a story. The BDAE "Cookie Theft" picture descriptions appearing in Figs. 8.4 and 8.5 are examples of narrative writing. These attempts to describe the events taking place in the picture provide us with rich information regarding the patient's graphomotor, written word-finding, spelling, and syntactic skills. The use of a standard picture is strongly recommended for both verbal and written descriptions because it allows us to compare patients to one another and to themselves over several testing sessions. For a shorter sample, in the absence of a picture, we might ask the patient to write a full sentence describing his vocation or the weather.

VI. Evaluating Reading Skills

A. Basic Concepts in Testing

It is not unusual for the inexperienced clinician to assess reading comprehension mistakenly on the basis of oral reading skills when in fact the ability to read aloud may be dissociated from the ability to comprehend the written word. To illustrate this point, consider that if you were presented with foreign words written in the Roman alphabet, you may be able to read them aloud without understanding their meaning (e.g., the Portuguese word *debandada*). You would merely verbalize the sounds associated with the letters without reference to their symbolic value. Conversely, you may have a store of written words that you can read for meaning but have never heard pronounced aloud. For example, you might know the meaning of the word *segue* without knowing how to pronounce it.

In all tests of reading, the clinician should attend carefully to errors as well as correct responses and choices. It is important to note, for example, whether the patient makes semantic substitution errors (e.g. "pond"/*lake*) or phonemic errors ("sleet"/*sleep*). The former may be indicative of **deep dyslexia** or of right-hemispheric processing of the material. These observations may be important from a theoretical and therapeutic perspective.

Remember: When testing reading skills in aphasia, tasks of reading aloud should be differentiated from tasks of reading for comprehension. The clinician should not speak globally of "reading" skills when referring just to oral reading.

B. Reading Aloud

When testing the ability to read aloud, one should have a variety of material available. Typically, the easiest materials are highly familiar, single words (e.g., the patient's first name) or words with emotional value (e.g., *blood*). Just as differences may be seen in patients' ability to repeat nouns, verbs, numbers, letters, grammatical words, and so forth, differences may be seen in the ability to read these various types of stimuli aloud. If the patient shows some ability to read single words aloud, then sentences varying in length and semantic, phonemic, and grammatical complexity should be offered. As in all tasks, record the exact nature of the patient's responses because they may form the basis of a therapy program.

C. Reading Comprehension

There are several ways to test reading comprehension in aphasia. Perhaps the best way to evaluate comprehension at the single-word level is to have the patient match printed words with pictorial representations of these words. It is possible also to get a sense of whether a word has been comprehended by noting the patient's reaction to it. For example, one of the words chosen for the *Boston Assessment of Severe Aphasia* is *Hitler,* because even though some patients cannot read this word aloud, they may show through negative reactions that its meaning is appreciated. Similarly, some patients may indicate understanding by showing the "Heil Hitler" salute when the word is presented, and many are able to match this word with the swastika symbol.

To test general appreciation of semantic class, the examiner can engage the patient in an "odd man out" task, which involves presenting a list of words in which one word does not belong (e.g., carrots, peas, *roses,* potatoes). The patient is required merely to indicate his or her choices. Similarly, a long list of items may be presented to see if the patient can group words according to semantic class (e.g., tools, clothing, furniture).

To test comprehension of sentence-length material, one can turn to sentence completion tasks in which the patient selects the best ending from among alternatives (e.g. "We write on a blackboard with ____." 1. pencils 2. chalk 3. erasers 4. slate). Reading more complex passages is assessed by asking the patient to select the phrase or sentence that best captures the meaning of the paragraph.

Perhaps the least successful approach to testing reading comprehension in aphasia is to ask the patient to follow written commands (e.g., "Pick up the pen"). Many patients have great difficulty understanding the purpose of such a task, as we rarely encounter such written commands in daily life. Sometimes, however, when a patient demonstrates profound auditory comprehension difficulties, such as those seen in the syndrome of Wernicke's aphasia or pure word deafness, one does test the ability to follow written commands. If such a patient can understand and follow written (but not spoken) commands, this finding has implications for management.

VII. Assessing Automatized Speech and Singing

In addition to the many propositional speech tasks undertaken during the language examination, automatized speech and singing should be assessed. Among the reasons for this are that (a) severely aphasic patients may produce real words only when reciting overlearned sequences or when singing familiar songs, (b) patients with transcortical motor aphasia may perform these tasks so well their performance stands in stark contrast to that seen on other verbal output tasks, and (c) complete failure to "carry a tune" may be indicative of right-hemisphere involvement.

A. Automatized Sequences

Overlearned verbal tasks include serial recitation of numbers, letters of the alphabet, days of the week, and months of the year. Because serial counting is probably the most robust of these tasks, if undertaken first it may induce perseveration that contaminates subsequent performance. For example, patients who have counted to 10 before trying to recite the days of the week may go on to say, "Monday, Tuesday, Threesday, Foursday . . . ." On the other hand, the months of the year may be particularly difficult; if undertaken first, they can cause frustration and subsequently poor performance on other rote tasks. For these reasons, the present authors use the following order when testing recitation of automatized sequences: days of the week, counting, alphabet, and months of the year.

Another form of automatic speech is recitation of overlearned materials such as prayers, poems, and nursery rhymes. The choice of these materials will vary according to the patient's background. Most Americans are familiar with "Mary Had a Little Lamb," "Hickory, Dickory, Dock," or the "Pledge of Allegiance," while Christians may easily recite the "Lord's Prayer."

The goal for all tests of automatized speech tasks is to elicit a run of speech from the patient. To accomplish this, the clinician may need to get the patient started and provide occasional cues when his or her performance begins to deteriorate.

B. Singing

In testing singing skills, the ability to produce a correct tune should be distinguished from the ability to produce words in song. For this reason, begin by asking the patient to hum or merely "dum-dum" the tune of a familiar song before adding the words. Among Americans, "Happy Birthday" and the national anthem are among the most familiar songs, but choices beyond these two may depend upon the patient's age and background. Older patients, for example, do very well with "Down by the Old Mill Stream" and "I've Been Workin' on the Railroad." Begin the singing task by saying "Let's hum some songs. Do you know ____? How does it go?" If the patient cannot initiate the tasks, the clinician can start out in unison and then fade his or her support, cueing along the way if required. After assessing the tune the patient produces in humming, ask him or her to sing the words. Some patients have a remarkable ability to produce correct words only in the context of a song and prove to be good candidates for Melodic Intonation Therapy (see chapter 15). Others, such as those with Wernicke's aphasia, may be able to hum a tune, but when they attempt to add words, the tune is destroyed by paraphasias. Patients who are not able to produce a tune under any circumstances may have right-hemisphere involvement, and this possibility should be explored with other forms of testing.

(Diagnoses based on speech samples on p. 109: Sample 1, Wernicke's aphasia; Sample 2, Broca's aphasia; Sample 3, transcortical motor aphasia.)

References and Suggested Readings

Goodglass, H., & Kaplan, E. (1984). *Boston Diagnostic Aphasia Examination.* Philadelphia: Lea & Febiger.

Helm-Estabrooks, N. (1991). *Aphasia Diagnostic Profiles.* San Antonio, TX: Special Press.

Helm-Estabrooks, N., Gress, C., & Sperry, E. (in press). *Scales of Language Comprehension.* San Antonio, TX: Special Press.

Helm-Estabrooks, N., Ramsberger, G., Morgan, A., & Nicholas, M. (1989). *Boston Assessment of Severe Aphasia.* San Antonio, TX: Special Press.

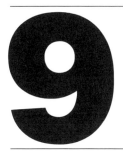

Apraxia Examination

In neurobehavioral terms, the word *praxis* refers to the ability to produce purposive movements. *Apraxia,* then, refers to a disturbance in the ability to produce purposive movement despite intact mobility. More precisely, apraxia is defined as an inability (or compromised ability) to program, sequence, and execute purposeful gestures, either on command or in imitation, subsequent to brain damage. Apraxia *cannot* be accounted for by loss of strength, feeling, or muscle coordination, or by confusion or inattention; instead, it is diagnosed only if the patient understands the task and possesses the physical capacity to perform the gestures but fails to execute the gesture in a normal manner (Geschwind, 1975). The often used term **ideomotor apraxia** attempts to capture this phenomenon by indicating that it is the "idea" of the motor aspects of the gesture that is disturbed.

In addition to ideomotor apraxia, two other terms are commonly used: **limb kinetic apraxia** and **ideational apraxia**. Currently, doubt exists as to whether limb kinetic apraxia can be distinguished from the motor signs of mild paresis. Ideational apraxia is a higher level disorder in which the individual movements are intact but the execution of complex sequential movements with objects is impaired (e.g., the patient tries to smoke the match instead of the cigarette). Many investigators consider ideational apraxia a severe form of ideomotor apraxia, or perhaps the result of generalized confusion. Because of the uncertainty surrounding limb kinetic and ideational apraxia, the following discussion will concentrate on ideomotor apraxia, a widely accepted and frequently occurring disorder within the aphasic population.

There are two major forms of ideomotor apraxia: **limb ideomotor apraxia** and **oral ideomotor apraxia**. (Although it will be dropped at this point for purposes of economy, the term *ideomotor* is implied throughout the following discussion.) **Limb apraxia** involves movements of nonparalyzed fingers, wrist, elbow, and shoulder. **Oral apraxia** involves movements of the oral/respiratory structures. The patient with apraxia can produce normal limb or oral movements reflexively or in the context of daily activities, but cannot upon command or in imitation. Thus, when instructed to "pretend you are combing your hair" or when given a model of the action, the apraxic patient has difficulty in executing an acceptable gesture. This difficulty can range from a mild awkwardness, fumbling, or self-correction to the absence of the most basic components of the gestures (e.g., simply pointing to his or her head to represent combing).

Remember: Sometimes severely apraxic patients have difficulty manipulating and using real objects in natural settings, but clinically apraxia refers to an impairment in the ability to produce purposeful gestures upon command or by imitation.

I. Implications of Apraxia

Apraxia commonly is associated with damage of the left cerebral hemisphere and therefore may coexist with aphasia. Apraxia and aphasia are not necessarily correlated with one another, so it is difficult to predict performance on an aphasia examination on the basis of performance on an apraxia examination. Despite this general truth, severe limb apraxia often is associated with limited ability to communicate gesturally, and severe oral apraxia often is associated with restricted verbal expression. When oral apraxia coexists with impaired ability to target speech sounds voluntarily, a diagnosis of **apraxia of speech** is used by some investigators. (In our clinic, the term is not commonly applied as a diagnostic label because patients with oral/speech apraxia typically have language deficits that lend themselves to classification according to the aphasia diagnosis system described in preceding chapters.) For more information on apraxia of speech, the reader is referred to Wertz, LaPointe, and Rosenbek (1984).

Severe apraxia of any form can affect the clinical evaluation process because all tests (including audiological, language, and cognitive examinations) require the patient to produce purposeful movements. In the extreme, the patient with severe oral and limb apraxia will have no reliable, purposeful output pathway. Such a patient, for example, may be incapable of reliably isolating and extending his index finger for pointing, shaking his head "yes" and "no," or saying these words. This degree of apraxia will affect the assessment of auditory comprehension and of verbal and graphic skills. It also will interfere with the neuropsychological assessment of intelligence and memory. Finally, severe apraxia may compromise the use of symbolic gestures for purposes of daily communication.

Remember: Apraxia can interfere with language and cognitive test performance and functional communication. An early apraxia examination, therefore, is of crucial importance in the assessment of the aphasic patient.

II. Varieties of Apraxia

A. Limb Apraxia

Limb apraxia can be viewed according to (a) which part of the hand/arm is most involved in the movement, (b) whether a pretended tool or instrument is associated with the movement, and (c) whether the locus of the movement is on the body or away from the body. Each of these ways of looking at limb apraxia should be considered separately:

1. **Distal versus proximal gestures.** There is evidence that the gross movements of the shoulder, arm, and fingers are subserved by a phylogenetically (evolution of the species) older **proximal motor system**, and the finer movements of the hand and fingers are subserved by a phylogenetically newer **distal motor system**. Apraxia, as a disorder of learned, representational movements, may effect the phylogenetically newer distal movements to a greater extent than the older proximal movements. Therefore, in evaluating apraxia the clinician should test both proximal gestures (e.g., pretending to hail a cab) and distal gestures (e.g., making the "V" for "victory"), beginning with proximal movements.

2. **Intransitive versus transitive gestures.** Proximal and distal gestures can be subdivided further according to whether a pretended tool or instrument is involved in the action. **Intransitive gestures** do not involve tool use (e.g., waving goodbye [proximal intransitive], making the "okay" sign [distal intransitive]). **Transitive gestures** are those requiring pretended tool use (e.g., painting a ceiling [proximal transitive], using a hand calculator [distal tran-

sitive]). Commonly, intransitive gestures are easier than transitive gestures, just as proximal gestures are easier than distal gestures.

3. **On the body versus away from body gestures.** The final subdivision for limb gestures is based on the locus of the action; that is to say, whether the locus of the movement is on the patient's body (e.g., brushing one's own hair) or whether it is away from the patient's body (e.g., brushing a dog). For many patients, away-from-the-body gestures are easier to perform than on-the-body gestures.

Thus one can see that in examining a patient for limb apraxia, the clinician should choose items that involve whole arm and shoulder (proximal) movement as well as those involving hand and fine finger (distal) movement. Within these subcategories some items should not require pretended use of a tool (intransitive) and some should require the pretended use of a tool (transitive). Finally, some items in each subcategory should take place on the body and some should be directed away from the body.

As a general rule, most patients with limb apraxia will show the least difficulty performing proximal, intransitive gestures away from the body (e.g., waving goodbye) and the greatest difficulty performing distal, transitive gestures on the body (e.g., tweezing eyebrows).

B. Oral Apraxia

The first important subclassification of gestures used in testing oral apraxia is whether the respiratory apparatus is involved. If the target gesture is independent of respiration (e.g., licking an ice cream cone), it is called a **nonrespiratory oral gesture**. If the target gesture involves inhalation or exhalation (e.g., blowing out a candle), it is labeled a **respiratory oral gesture**. Most patients with oral apraxia will experience greater difficulty performing respiratory than nonrespiratory gestures.

Like limb gestures, oral gestures can be further subdivided according to whether or not a pretended tool is involved. An example of an intransitive oral gesture is smiling; sipping through a straw is an example of a transitive oral gesture. Typically, intransitive oral gestures are easier than transitive oral gestures. Further, most patients with oral apraxia will show the least difficulty in producing intransitive nonrespiratory movements (e.g., smiling) and the greatest difficulty performing respiratory transitive movements (e.g., sniffing a flower).

III. Testing for Apraxia

All aphasic patients should be tested for the presence and severity of apraxia, with the examination of limb apraxia preceding that of oral apraxia because limb gestures tend to be easier. Begin by telling the patient that he or she will be asked to do some things without talking. Then, after indicating (by touching) the patient's nonhemiplegic hand/arm, say "Use your hand and show me how you would pretend to _____." (If possible, both hands should be tested.) If the patient seems not to have understood the command, then provide further contextual cues (e.g., "Sometimes your hair gets messy [pointing to the patient's hair] and you have to comb it. Pretend you have a comb and show me how you would comb your hair"). If the patient still has done nothing to indicate that he or she has understood the command, present the gesture for imitation (e.g., "Pretend to comb your hair like this"). Because auditory comprehension must be adequate to understand verbal commands, some clinicians test apraxia only by imitation. However, it is important to determine, if possible, the patient's ability to self-generate a symbolic movement. Therefore, the "to command" condition should be attempted in all cases. In many cases, the patient produces enough of the target movement to indicate an understanding of the command. If the performance is not within normal limits, the full set of gestures should be repeated for imitation after all have been given to command. The test hierarchy for limb gestures is presented in Table 9.1.

After the limb apraxia exam has been completed both to command and by imitation, prepare the patient for the oral apraxia exam with the instruction, "Now I want you to do some things with your mouth and face (touch the patient's cheek), but again, no talking." Do not allow the patient to self-cue with hand gestures. The test hierarchy for oral gestures is presented in Table 9.2.

IV. Praxis Response Types

Although each apraxic patient has the potential of producing a unique response, certain responses are commonly observed in examining praxis skills and these can be discussed in a somewhat

TABLE 9.1
Limb Apraxia Test Hierarchy

Limb gesture	Test
PROXIMAL	**"Show me how you would pretend to . . ."**
Intransitive	
Away from body	". . . wave goodbye."
On body	". . . wipe your brow as if hot."
Transitive	
Away from body	". . . paint the ceiling."
	". . . jack up a car."
On body	". . . brush your hair."
DISTAL	**"Show me how you would . . ."**
Intransitive	
Away from body	". . . make the 'okay' sign."
	". . . thumb a ride."
On body	". . . tap your forehead as if thinking."
Transitive	
Away from body	". . . flip a coin."
	". . . tap a telegraph key."
On body	". . . tweeze your eyebrows."

hierarchical order, beginning with the most impaired. If the patient produces a response that cannot be captured by this classification system, the clinician should record the exact response. This information may be useful both in understanding the nature of the disorder and in planning treatment programs.

A. No Response (NR)

There are several reasons why a patient may fail to respond to a task, among them being the possibility that the patient (a) is not cognitively alert, (b) is not in the "set" for the task, (c) does not understand the verbal command, or (d) is uncooperative. The clinician must determine which of these (or some other) factors accounts for the failure to respond. One then should try to elicit a response from the patient by providing further instruction or even contextual cues, such as showing him or her the desired gesture and asking for imitation.

TABLE 9.2
Oral Apraxia Test Hierarchy

Oral gesture	Test
NONRESPIRATORY	**"Show me how you would . . ."**
Intransitive	". . . smile."
	". . . kiss."
Transitive	". . . lick an ice cream cone."
	". . . bite an apple."
RESPIRATORY	**"Show me how you would . . ."**
Intransitive	". . . whistle."
	". . . cough."
	". . . sniff a strange smell."
Transitive	". . . sip through a straw."
	". . . blow out a birthday cake."
	". . . smoke a cigarette."

B. Diffuse Movement (DM)

The patient may simply wave his or her hand or move the mouth in a diffuse or meaningless way. In these cases, the previously listed methods for eliciting a better performance are used.

C. Verbal Response (VR)

Instead of producing a gestural response, the patient may produce a verbal response that represents the action (e.g., says "Blow, blow" instead of blowing).

D. Perseverative Response (PR)

Patients often produce part or all of a previous gesture, referred to as perseveration. This phenomenon is more likely to occur if the presentation of stimuli is too rapid or if insufficient attention has been given to establishing set. Perseverative responses are less likely to occur when the patient is imitating a clinician's model than when he or she is responding to verbal commands. When perseveration does occur, the testing should proceed more slowly, with increased latencies between items and the instruction, "Now here is a new one. Show me how . . . ."

E. Deictic Gesture (DG)

Within this category, the patient simply points to the locus of the action (e.g., to his nose for "sniffing"; to the ceiling for "painting the ceiling"). When deictic responses occur, the clinician should provide verbal reinforcement and restate the instruction (e.g., "That's right, you do it with your nose, but can you sniff as if something smells bad?").

F. Parapractic Gesture (PP)

In this instance the patient substitutes a semantically related, nonperseverative gesture for another (e.g., sawing a board instead of pounding a nail, even though the patient has understood the command). This is the gestural counterpart to a verbal/semantic paraphasia in which one word is substituted for a related word (e.g. "saw"/*hammer*). As with the verbal paraphasias, the patient may be able to self-correct a parapractic error if it is called to his or her attention.

G. Body Part as Object (BPO)

This error is seen only in testing transitive gestures. The patient in this case uses part of his or her body (usually the hand or fingers) as the pretended object (e.g., combs hair with fingers instead of pretending to hold a comb; stirs coffee with finger instead of pretending to hold a spoon). In such cases, the clinician should give further instruction (e.g., "That's right, but you're using your fingers. Can you pretend you're holding a comb?"). If this is unsuccessful, provide a model for imitation.

H. Holding Minus Movement (H–M)

This error, too, is seen only in testing transitive gestures. In this instance, the patient pretends to hold the object of the action (e.g., a toothbrush), but fails to produce the movement (e.g., brushing). When the H–M error occurs, verbally encourage the patient to produce the movement before imitation is attempted.

I. Holding with Diffuse Movement (HDM)

Characteristic of this response, the patient pretends to hold and move the object, but the movement is diffuse and lacks the essential elements for the target gesture. In such cases one would ask, "Can you do it better? Show me how you brush your teeth."

J. Holding, Correct Movement but Minus Extent of the Object (H–EO)

In this error type, the patient pretends to hold the object and makes a correct gesture, but he or she fails to represent the extent or size of the object (e.g., pretends to hold toothbrush and brush teeth but holds clenched hand next to teeth).

K. Holding, Correct Movement and Correct Extent of the Object (H + EO)

This response is the normal, correct production of a transitive movement.

If the clinician wishes to assign scores to each of the gestural responses, in order to quantify the patient's praxic skills, the following scoring system based on Helm-Estabrooks (1991) may be used:

3 (Normal). Performance is within normal limits for the dominant or nondominant hand. There is no notable hesitancy, fumbling, or self-correction. In the case of transitive movements, the performance is classified as H + EO (holding, correct movement and correct extent of the object).

2 (Adequate). The patient may hesitate or self-correct his or her performance, or the movement may lack sharpness although the crucial components of the gesture are present (e.g., stirring coffee without allowing for the correct length of the spoon handle). In the case of transitive movements, the performance may be classified as H–EO (holding, correct movement but minus the extent of the object).

1 (Partially Adequate). Some basic components of the target response are retained, but the patient uses a body part as the object (BPO; e.g., brushing teeth with forefinger) or the object is represented by a "holding" posture, though movement is diffuse (HDM) or absent (H–M).

0 (Inadequate). The response lacks any of the crucial components of the target movement—sawing instead of hammering (parapractic gesture), saying "Cough, cough" instead of coughing (verbal response), pointing to the lips for kissing (deictic gesture), producing a previous gesture from a previous response (perseverative response), producing only a diffuse movement (DM), or failing to respond (NR).

References and Suggested Readings

Geschwind, N. (1975). The apraxias: Neural mechanisms of disorders of learned movement. *American Scientist, 63*(2), 188–195.

Helm-Estabrooks, N. (1991). *Test of Oral and Limb Apraxia.* San Antonio, TX: Special Press.

Wertz, R.T., LaPointe, L., & Rosenbek, J.C. (1984). *Apraxia of speech in adults: The disorder and its management.* New York: Grune & Stratton.

Section Three

**Implementing
Aphasia Therapy and
Measuring Its Effects**

10

Using the Process Approach to Generate Treatment Programs

As described throughout the preceding discussion, meaningful information about a patient's behavior comes from a careful description and analysis of exactly what he or she did while trying to arrive at a correct response. In contrast to emphasizing final scores, this process approach tells the clinician about the patient's strengths, weaknesses, strategies, and compensatory behaviors—the foundation on which to generate hypotheses and build aphasia treatment programs.

I. Applying the Process Approach

A. Analyzing Responses to a Responsive Naming Task

One way of testing word-retrieval skills is to ask the patient a question such as "How many days are there in a week?" The following responses to this question were elicited from seven different patients:

1. "One, two, three, four, five, six, *seven.*"

2. Wrote "7" in the air.

3. "Beben."

4. Indicated seven with fingers.

5. "Six, no not six, one more."

6. "I know. Wait a minute. Days in a week. There are . . . there are seven days in a week."

7. "Seven."

All of the preceding responses indicate that the individuals knew how many days are in a week. Only patient 7, however, produced the correct word in immediate response to the question (unless one credits "beben" in patient 3, who had Broca's aphasia and dysarthria, and consistently replaced sibilant

147

sounds with bilabials). Patient 1 could not produce any isolated numbers (except *one*) but effectively counted up to the target. Patients 2 and 4 used meaningful gestures to communicate the message. Patient 5 never produced the word *seven* through any mode, but he nonetheless indicated by his circumlocutory response that he knew the answer to the question. Finally, patient 6 was slow, but ultimately successful, in retrieving and producing the answer "seven." The treatment approach in each case will differ according to the underlying problem and available strengths suggested by the nature of the response. Another important point to remember is that overall scores on tests with subparts can mask differences in patient performance, as will be illustrated in the next section.

Note: When recording patients' responses, checkmarks are used only when responses are immediately and fully correct. Otherwise, the actual response or behavior is recorded. This is true of both verbal and nonverbal responses.

B. Analyzing Responses to an Auditory Comprehension Task

Two patients received similar scores (27/72 vs. 26/72) on the Word Discrimination subtest of the *Boston Diagnostic Aphasia Examination* (see Figs. 10.1 and 10.2). Both patients quickly identified eight of the items, earning 2 points for each. On closer examination, however, one can see differences on the items that were immediately understood. Patient A earned full credit for three object names (*key, feather,* and *hammock*), one letter (*H*), one action word (*sleeping*), two colors (*red* and *purple*), and one number (*1936*). In contrast, patient B earned full credit for one object name (*glove*), one letter (*S*), three action words (*running, falling,* and *dripping*), one color (*blue*), and two numbers (*42* and *7000*). In addition to showing no agreement on the items that were immediately understood, the two patients revealed different patterns of strengths and weaknesses in comprehension within semantic categories (see Table 10.1). This observation has important implications for treatment, because the strengths can be used as "springboards" for rehabilitation.

If one of the treatment goals for patients A and B was to improve the comprehension of spoken single words, then for patient A the clinician might begin treatment with the rela-

Card 2 OBJECTS:	IDENTIFICATION Under 5 seconds 2 points	Over 5 seconds 1 point	CATE-GORY 1/2 point	CUE 1/2 point	FAIL 0	Card 3 ACTIONS:	IDENTIFICATION Under 5 seconds 2 points	Over 5 seconds 1 point	CATE-GORY 1/2 point	CUE 1/2 point	FAIL 0
chair	*hammock* →			✓		smoking	✓				
key	✓					drinking	*running*			✓	
glove	✓			✓		running	*dripping*			✓	
feather	✓					sleeping	✓				
hammock	✓					falling	*smoking*			*sleeping* ✓	
cactus				✓		dripping	*running*		✓		
LETTERS:						COLORS:					
L		*R*	✓			blue	*Smoking*			*red* ✓	
H	✓					brown	*blue*		✓		
R		*7*	✓			red	✓				
T		*L*	✓			pink	*brown*			✓	
S	*Spiral*			"T" ✓		gray	*Pink*			✓	
G	*Circle*			"R" ✓		purple	✓				
FORMS:						NUMBERS:					
circle	*Chair*			*Spiral* ✓		7			✓		
spiral	*T*			*Star* ✓		42			✓		
square	*Cactus*			*link* ✓		700	*7*	✓			
triangle	*. H*			*Cone* ✓		1936	✓				
cone	*Key* ✓			*Square* ✓		15		✓			
star	✓					7000	*7cv*			✓	

Raw Score: **27**

FIG. 10.1. Word Discrimination, Patient A (From *Boston Diagnostic Aphasia Examination* by Harold Goodglass and Edith Kaplan. Copyright 1984 by Lea & Febiger. Reprinted by permission.)

tively strong semantic categories of object and number names. These two categories then might be combined with numbers for improving the comprehension of phrases, as in "two apples." Later, patient A's third strongest category (colors) could be added, as in "three green apples" versus "two red apples."

In the case of patient B, who showed good ability to comprehend the names of actions, this category could be expanded to include actions that also are the names of objects (e.g., comb, iron). This approach may have a deblocking effect on his relatively poor ability to comprehend object names.

Let us now turn to another example of how the process approach to examination of language allows us to generate treatment programs.

Card 2 — IDENTIFICATION

OBJECTS:	Under 5 seconds — 2 points	Over 5 seconds — 1 point	CATE-GORY 1/2 point	CUE 1/2 point	FAIL 0
chair	key		✓		
key	L ✓			glove ✓	
glove	✓				
feather	triangle			key ✓	
hammock	square			glove ✓	
cactus	H			feather ✓	
LETTERS:					
L				✓	
H	chair			L ✓	
R	circle			S ✓	
T	square			H ✓	
S	✓				
G	hammock			H ✓	
FORMS:					
circle	"S"			spiral ✓	
spiral	H		✓		
square	key			circle ✓	
triangle	hammock			square ✓	
cone	H			square ✓	
star	chair			triangle ✓	

Card 3 — IDENTIFICATION

ACTIONS:	Under 5 seconds — 2 points	Over 5 seconds — 1 point	CATE-GORY 1/2 point	CUE 1/2 point	FAIL 0
smoking		✓			
drinking	falling		✓		
running	✓				
sleeping	brown				✓
falling	✓				
dripping	✓				
COLORS:					
blue	✓				
brown	pink			✓	
red	falling				✓
pink	red		✓		
gray	purple		✓		
purple	red		✓		
NUMBERS:					
7		✓			
42	✓				
700		✓			
1936		✓			
15	✓	✓			
7000	✓				

* NB. First letter of last name

Raw Score: 26

FIG. 10.2. Word Discrimination, Patient B (From *Boston Diagnostic Aphasia Examination* by Harold Goodglass and Edith Kaplan. Copyright 1984 by Lea & Febiger. Reprinted by Permission.)

C. Analyzing Responses to a Confrontation Naming Task

The *Boston Naming Test* (Kaplan, Goodlass, & Weintraub, 1984) is a commonly used assessment of confrontation naming skills. The following answers were elicited from six different patients presented with the target of a harmonica:

1. "A musical thing you blow through."

2. "A marhonika."

3. "Mon-ka."

4. "A frelicka."

5. "I know it but I can't say it."

6. "A double-decker bus."

TABLE 10.1
Patterns of Strength and Weakness in Similar Scores on a Word Discrimination Test

Semantic category	Patient A (points)	Patient B (points)
Objects	6.5	2.5
Numbers	6.0	8.0
Colors	5.5	4.5
Actions	4.5	8.0
Letters	3.5	2.5*
Forms	1.0**	.5
Total score:	27.0	26.0

*The only letter identified correctly by Patient B was *S,* which is the first letter of his last name. He did, however, earn an additional half-point for recognizing that *L* is a letter.

**Although he lost 1 point for slowness, Patient A identified the geometric form "star," which is also the name of an object (his strongest category). He failed to identify all other form names.

Although no patient named this item correctly, it would be wrong to state that all six had a word-finding problem. In fact, patient 6, who misperceived the stimulus (interpreting the two rows of air holes as windows and calling the object a "double-decker bus"), may not have had a word-finding problem at all. Similarly, patient 3 ("Mon-ka), who demonstrated great articulatory struggle, particularly on initially unstressed words, actually may have had good word-finding skills. Patient 1 ("A musical thing you blow through"), provided enough semantic information to suggest that he had formed appropriate associations for this item, and patient 2 ("A marhonika") provided enough phonemic information to suggest that he had a specific appropriate label in mind. Patient 4 ("A frelika") produced a multisyllable neologism (new word), the final syllable of which was correct, which offered only minimal evidence that he had a phonemic representation for the target word. Patient 5 ("I know it but I can't say it") failed to provide any semantic or phonological information about the word, suggesting profound word-retrieval problems.

All of these naming responses were incorrect and earned a score of zero. The patients who provided these responses had the following diagnoses: (1) anomic aphasia, (2) conduction aphasia, (3) Broca's aphasia, (4) Wernicke's aphasia, (5) anomic aphasia (of a more profound variety than #1), and (6) right-hemispheric stroke. Because these responses indicate differing underlying bases for the "naming problem" in each patient, it follows that the treatment approaches to these problems also will, or should, differ. A few examples may suffice in making this point.

In the case of patient 3 (Broca's aphasia), the deficient response probably was caused by articulatory struggle rather than word-finding difficulty. Such patients often have particular difficulty initiating words beginning with unvoiced sounds in unstressed syllables (as in the target *harmonica*) and perform better with words beginning with voiced sounds in stressed syllables (e.g., *banana*). Rather than working directly on word finding, which may not be the primary problem in this patient, the best therapeutic approach might be to improve articulation through a method such as Melodic Intonation Therapy (see chapter 15). Melodic Intonation Therapy facilitates articulation in patients with Broca's aphasia because each syllable is isolated and stressed with continuous voicing.

The response of patient 5 with severe anomic aphasia offered little evidence that he had access to the semantic associations that could lead to retrieval of the word *harmonica*. His treatment (unlike that for the patient with Broca's aphasia) may begin at a basic level of word retrieval, using a multimodal stimulation approach that employs concrete, picturable, emotionally laden objects that are associated with a distinct gesture (e.g., a gun). In contrast, patient 1 (with a milder form of anomia) demonstrated through his circumlocutory speech that he retained rich associations for the object (harmonica). Like many of us, he tried to cue himself by talking about the object while attempting to retrieve the exact label. Some of the therapeutic strategies that may be successful with a patient such as this include encouragement of descriptive circumlocutions, the use of representational gestures, and drawing (see chapter 13), all of which may stimulate word retrieval.

II. Hypotheses for Aphasia Treatment Programs

The preceding examples were drawn from responses to standardized language tests. It should be noted, however, that the clinician often must venture outside the realm of a formally administered aphasia test in order to plan and carry out an appropriate treatment program. Testing limb and bucco/facial praxis skills (see chapter 9), for example, is essential, as is the assessment of visuospatial and visual memory skills (see chapter 7). In addition, the results of the neurologic examination (see chapter 4) are extremely important to the speech clinician. In fact, *only an interdisciplinary approach* to the assessment of the aphasia patient provides the crucial information regarding the integrity or impairment of skill areas essential to the rehabilitation of communicative function. All clinicians have an obligation to note the processes and strategies the patient is using to arrive at a solution or response. With this information one can hypothesize as to which underlying brain mechanisms and behaviors are retained and which are damaged. This information then helps generate the hypothesis that forms the basis of treatment.

A. Hypothesis

This patient *is not* performing correctly in this sphere because _____, but he does have the potential for correct performance as demonstrated by _____.

As stated, in order to generate this hypothesis one must study this patient's behavior, noting exactly what he does both within and outside the testing environment. For example, recently Mr. C was referred for assessment 24 years after a stroke that followed open heart surgery at age 38. The *Boston Diagnostic Aphasia Examination* (BDAE) was administered, and his auditory comprehension was found relatively well preserved. On all verbal tasks, however, his output was limited to "yes" and "no"; single syllables were produced with a great amount of groping as he tried ineffectively to control his articulators. Mr. C could not communicate through writing, but he spontaneously used some gestures to convey meaning (e.g., when asked "What do you do with a razor?" he pantomimed shaving). Similarly, when shown the "NO SMOKING" sign on the *Boston Assessment of Severe Aphasia* (BASA), he pantomimed smoking and then gestured "no." On the relatively easier BASA he was unable to perform any verbal task beyond answering "yes" or "no"; however, he was able to match written words correctly with pictures and objects. On the *Boston Apraxia Test* (see chapter 9) he demonstrated only mild bucco/facial apraxia.

The only time Mr. C was heard to produce real words (beyond the unreliable production of "yes" and "no") was during the BDAE auditory Word Discrimination subtest, when he easily articulated the words *here, water,* and *shoe* as he pointed to pictures (however, *water* and *shoe* are not stimuli on this test). The examiner hypothesized that this patient failed all BDAE and BASA verbal tasks because he no longer could articulate words voluntarily or purposefully. He was, however, capable of incidental speech during a nonverbal task.

B. Application of the Hypothesis

Mr. C did not produce real words on any verbal task because of an impairment in the voluntary control of speech. He has a capacity for producing real words, however, as evidenced by the incidental speech he produced during an auditory comprehension task.

The therapeutic task in this case becomes one of using Mr. C's spared ability to produce incidental speech to deblock his impaired ability to produce purposeful speech. In BASA and BDAE testing, the examiner noted that although Mr. C did not produce real words for the written stimuli in the oral reading tasks, he had some preserved ability to read single words for meaning, matching them accurately to pictures and objects. What if his own, involuntarily produced words were presented to him in written form? If these words held some meaning for him and if he could read them aloud, could they be brought under more voluntary control for verbal expression and used propositionally? This, then, was the therapeutic experiment, which showed that indeed he could read two of the three words aloud. Furthermore, when shown pictures representing *water* and *shoe* he could name them.

The clinician then set about expanding Mr. C's lexicon. The only other words he had spoken during BDAE and BASA testing were "yes" and "no." He struggled to read these aloud, so these words were set aside and the clinician turned instead to words that were highly emotional and configural (containing some lowercase letters with ascenders and descenders). This decision was based on experimental evidence that words with these characteristics are easier for aphasic patients to read.

After creating a list of configural, emotional words, the clinician explained to Mr. C that she was presenting him with single words. He was not to struggle in his attempt to read these aloud but simply to utter the first thing that came to his lips (a difficult request of someone who had been struggling with speech for 24 years). If he read the word correctly, the clinician printed it on a 3″ × 5″ card. If it was a picturable word, she drew a picture of the target on the reverse side for confrontation naming. If he uttered another real word for the written target presented, the clinician discarded the original target and wrote down his word instead, to see if he could produce the word again voluntarily as a correct, propositional response. Using this approach, 20 words were presented in the first session. Of these, Mr. C read three aloud correctly with little or no struggle. These, like his original two words, were written on individual 3″ × 5″ index cards with their pictorial representation on the backs. He was given these cards for practice. In the next session Mr. C added three more words out of 20 new stimuli, and in the third session three more, one of which he had not been able to read aloud in the second session. At that point he could use the first nine words quite reliably for confrontation naming without first orally reading them. By the 10th session Mr. C's list looked like the following:

12/21/87	fish	tea	coffee	shoe	water		
12/22/87	ball	mother	ship				
12/24/87	cat	love	milk	home			
12/29/87	bus	car	horse				
12/31/87	father	two	sun	one	three		
1/4/88	fifty	Pat					
1/5/88	hat	eyes	fit	wise			
1/8/88	cop	form	pit	cow	hi	hay	ant
1/11/88	wash						
1/15/88	hand	pee					

Remember that the word choices were determined primarily by Mr. C. That is, although the clinician chose the words used to stimulate speech production, any real word he could read aloud was added to his list without regard to its functionality. Surprisingly, however, the list contains many functionally useful words.

Using the same line of reasoning described in the case of Mr. C, Helm and Barresi (1980) tried this approach with a 59-year-old stroke patient. Mr. L was 4 months post onset when we undertook this method, now called Voluntary Control of Involuntary Utterances or VCIU for short (see chapter 14). Before beginning VCIU, Mr. L had a profile of spared and impaired skills similar to that of Mr. C, except that this patient could read aloud and repeat a few BDAE words. At time of discharge he had a lexicon of 290 words that he could use propositionally for purposes of communication. Changes in BDAE performance were dramatic. Furthermore, once voluntary speech was deblocked his family reported continued progress at home.

Note: Some patients have similar profiles of spared and impaired abilities and similar problem-solving strategies. This means one does not necessarily have to develop a new and unique treatment program for each patient. A program that is successful with one patient having a certain performance profile may be successful with another showing the same constellation of strengths, weaknesses, and strategies.

Another choice of treatment for patients with severely restricted verbal output is Melodic Intonation Therapy (MIT). Good candidates for MIT are dysarthric and demonstrate substantial bucco/facial apraxia. Although Mr. C and Mr. L both had severely restricted verbal output, when they did produce words they articulated clearly, and bucco/facial praxis was relatively well preserved. Furthermore, Mr. C and Mr. L were not able to produce more words when singing popular songs, as good MIT candidates do. In fact, a trial of MIT was unsuccessful with Mr. L, and further exploration of the conditions under which he was able to produce real words led to the development of VCIU.

In describing the two patients above we have tried to demonstrate how the application of the process approach to the evaluation of language and related behaviors can produce the information necessary for developing appropriate treatment plans. Of course, it is expected that in some cases the results of the examination will suggest more than one approach to treatment. For example, a patient with severely restricted verbal output and relatively preserved auditory comprehension on examination may demonstrate some ability to produce words in song and to represent concepts through drawing. In such a case, a course of MIT may be combined with a drawing program, to facilitate return of functional communication. As each of these approaches is undertaken, the clinician should continue to use a process approach in evaluating the patient's responses to the treatment methods themselves and to the tests used to evaluate generalization effects.

References and Suggested Readings

Helm, N., & Barresi, B. (1980). Voluntary Control of Involuntary Utterances: A treatment approach for severe aphasia. In R. Brookshire (Ed.), *Clinical Aphasiology Conference Proceedings*. Minneapolis, MN: BRK.

Kaplan, E., Goodglass, H., & Weintraub, S. (1984). *The Boston Naming Test*. Philadelphia: Lea & Febiger.

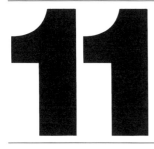

Measuring Treatment Effects

The goal of aphasia rehabilitation is to improve the patient's communication skills to a level beyond that which might be reached solely through the process referred to as **spontaneous recovery**. Spontaneous recovery is the period during which structurally undamaged portions of the brain (temporarily influenced by such factors as edema and local abnormalities of blood flow and metabolism) regain function. As a general rule, the greatest amount of spontaneous recovery occurs during the first 6 to 8 weeks after a stroke, although considerable variation may be seen depending on the stroke's etiology and the size of the lesion. Of course, some patients regain very little function through natural processes. In these cases especially, early intervention may prevent the development of negative behaviors that can become so entrenched that later attempts at treatment are unsuccessful.

To illustrate this point, consider a patient (Mr. K) referred for his first course of treatment 1 year after his stroke. When admitted for aphasia rehabilitation, Mr. K's speech output was limited to the nonsense stereotypy "bee-bah," which he produced with a range of emotional and intonational variations. Despite the fact that Mr. K could not communicate verbally, his family never asked him to produce a meaningful gesture, to write a few letters of key words, or to draw a picture, all of which he could do with encouragement. Instead, they bombarded him with questions (e.g., "What do you want? Are you hungry? Do you want to go somewhere?"), seldom asking the key question, so that mutual feelings of frustration often escalated to an explosive interchange. After a year of this negative behavior it was difficult to implement a successful treatment program.

Early intervention probably would have prevented this unfortunate situation. First, there are methods (e.g., Melodic Intonation Therapy) that may eliminate a nonsense stereotypy. Second, this patient had several channels of nonverbal expression that should have been encouraged as soon as it became obvious that he could not communicate verbally. Third, family counseling, along with an understanding of Mr. K's full range of skills, may have established a more positive communication environment.

In addition to experiencing great difficulty in communicating during the early weeks after stroke, many patients experience depression and feelings of loss, confusion, and isolation. A knowledgeable and caring clinician, using a well-conceived and well-implemented treatment program, can have a significant, positive impact during this difficult period. In addition, increasing health care costs and accountability demand that clinicians provide concrete evidence that their treatments have made a significant difference in their patients' recovery. This state of affairs has led to numerous group studies of treatment efficacy (e.g., see Shewan [1986] and Rosenbek, LaPointe, & Wertz [1989] for comprehensive reviews of this literature). In general, group studies are carried out by researchers; practicing clinicians, however, must approach each patient as a case study. For this reason, emphasis currently is placed on single-subject designs for measuring treatment effects in aphasia.

I. Measuring Treatment Effects in the Individual Patient

A. Dependent and Independent Variables

In order to show that the effects of treatment are significant, the clinician first must choose a treatment approach with a scoring system and a target behavior that can be measured by a test or some other reliable method. Both of these decisions then become variables in the treatment process and its measurement.

The **independent variable** is the variable manipulated by the clinician; it is the **treatment method**. The **dependent variable** is the variable affected by this manipulation; in aphasia, this is a disordered behavior (e.g., auditory comprehension) usually measured by a **test**.

When graphing a patient's response to treatment, the horizontal line represents the independent variable (the treatment method) across time, whereas the vertical line represents the measures of the dependent behavior (the test scores). An example of this is presented in Fig. 11.1. In this case the *Boston Naming Test* was administered after every 10 sessions of a therapy designed to improve naming in an anomic patient.

A common error made by less experienced clinicians centers around the belief that if a patient is making progress within a treatment program (the independent variable), then that program is effective. Instead, the effectiveness of a program is

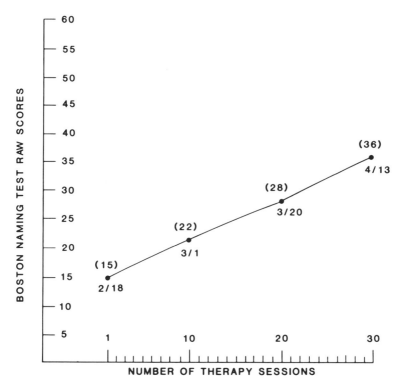

FIG. 11.1. A measurement of treatment response (administration date appears below raw score achieved)

measured according to progress documented for both the treatment (independent variable) and the target behavior as measured by a test (dependent variable). A good example is found in the Melodic Intonation Therapy study by Naeser and Helm-Estabrooks (1985). All eight patients studied were successful in completing the MIT program; that is, they improved on the independent variable as measured by scores earned from session to session. However, four of the patients showed no change in conversational speech skills; they did not improve on the dependent measure, the BDAE Conversational Speech scale. In other words, MIT was a successful method for only half the patients studied, even though all eight completed the program. Studying lesion sites in those with good and poor treatment response further delineated the characteristics of the optimal candidate for MIT (i.e., the patient who is likely both to complete the program and to show positive changes in conversational speech). This brings the discussion to a basic principle of treatment:

Note: It is the clinician's duty to discover the best way to help an aphasic patient. If a patient does not respond to a particular treatment program, other methods must be explored. If all best attempts to treat the patient fail, then the clinician must explore ways in which communicative factors external to the patient can be manipulated. Aphasic patients who seek our help do not fail us, but we sometimes fail them because our methods for treating brain damage are limited.

This manual discusses the use of the process approach for developing new treatment techniques or choosing from existing methods based on individual patient profiles (see chapter 10). In all cases, the clinician must determine a way of measuring both within-treatment response and generalization of the target skills. For example, when developing the program called Treatment of Aphasic Perseveration (TAP; see chapter 17), the present authors had to devise a scoring system that would allow the clinician to rate naming responses, so that the target stimuli could be hierarchically arranged. Each session then could begin with the stimuli most likely to elicit correct naming and least likely to elicit perseveration. This scoring system also was used to measure progress in TAP across sessions.

Measuring generalization of skills developed with TAP entailed choosing a test that would measure changes in the target skill (naming) and in the negative behavior (perseveration) manifested by some patients when they attempted to name. The BDAE Confrontation Naming subtest was chosen because it allows charting both increases in naming and decreases in perseveration as a result of treatment. In addition, performance on this subtest correlates significantly with the BDAE Aphasia Severity Rating, which is based in conversational and narrative speech performance (Goodglass & Kaplan, 1984). Furthermore, because the Confrontation Naming subtest is short, the clinician can readminister it after every 5 to 10 sessions of TAP. If no improvement is seen (at least qualitatively) on the dependent measure, one should reconsider the merits of the TAP program for a particular patient even if some progress is observed within the method itself.

B. Generalization of Treatment Effects

In choosing a test or subtest as the dependent measure of treatment effects, one does so in the hope that test performance represents or reflects the patient's ability to use these skills to communicate on a daily basis. It is not practical, however, to follow a patient around and observe him or her in a variety of communicative interactions. One turns instead to research evidence that performance on a particular test reflects communication ability in natural settings. Among the few such studies is that of Holland (1982), who observed patients in their natural environments and carefully noted all successful and unsuccessful attempts to communicate through speech, writing, gesturing, and so forth. At the same time, the patients were assessed with her *Communicative Abilities in Daily Living* (CADL; 1980). Holland found a strong, positive correlation between the two measures; that is, performance on the CADL did reflect communicative performance in natural environments. The clinician, therefore, can use the CADL with some confidence that improved post-therapy test scores are indicative of improved functional communication.

A different type of study was undertaken by Easterbrooks, Brown, and Perera (1982), who were interested in assessing the extent to which narrative descriptions of the BDAE "Cookie Theft" picture were reflective of conversational discourse skills. Five aphasic subjects were tested several times over a 1-year period. Comparisons of picture descriptions with conversational speech showed that the subjects produced a larger portion of discrete, grammatical, analyzable utterances in response to the picture, although a similar range and form of grammatical structures was elicited by the two conditions. Because of this parallel performance, Easterbrooks et al. suggest that the use of the "Cookie Theft" picture description is an economic way of predicting conversational speech skills. (The Easterbrooks et al. study also led Menn, Helm-Estabrooks, and Ramsberger [unpublished manuscript] to develop a method for more precisely analyzing "Cookie Theft" narratives, called the Communicative Effectiveness Profile, which is described in the latter part of this chapter.)

C. Single-Subject Designs

As mentioned previously, emphasis today is placed on single-subject designs for measuring the effects of aphasia therapy.

Three commonly used single-subject designs are the **multiple baseline design**, the **basic ABA or withdrawal design**, and the **alternating treatment design**. Brief discussions of each follow; for more in-depth descriptions, see Kearns (1986) and McReynolds and Thompson (1986).

1. **Multiple baseline design.** The multiple baseline design is recommended during the initial period post onset of aphasia, when spontaneous recovery is most likely to occur. In this design, performance on more than one target behavior is sampled throughout the course of treatment, but only one of the behaviors is treated. If treatment is successful, then presumably the treated behavior will improve significantly more than the untreated behaviors. Consider the following example.

   A patient with equally poor ability to name objects and actions on the BDAE Confrontation Naming subtest (the dependent measure) entered a program to improve object naming. Retesting at regular intervals showed that object naming steadily increased while action naming remained close to baseline. Although one might assume that the improvement was the result of treatment and not of spontaneous recovery, one problem with this assumption is that untreated behaviors likely have different patterns of recovery. For example, a longitudinal study by Fitzpatrick, Glosser, and Helm-Estabrooks (1988) found that repetition skills and auditory comprehension recovered significantly in the initial period post onset, whereas naming showed significant improvement in the later period. An additional challenge in interpreting the results of a multiple baseline study is that improvement on the treated behavior may generalize to performance on the untreated behavior. In fact, in the earlier example, the clinician might intentionally attempt to deblock action naming through the use of stimulus words such as *comb* and *milk* that denote both objects and actions. An alternative to the multiple baseline design is the basic ABA or withdrawal design.

2. **Basic ABA or withdrawal design.** In the basic ABA or withdrawal design, "A" is the **no treatment phase** and "B" is the **treatment phase**. First, a baseline performance is established by repeated testing of the dependent variable during the initial A phase. The patient then enters the

treatment or B phase and is retested. Treatment is subsequently withdrawn during the second A phase. If there is significantly improved test performance only during the B phase, that provides concrete evidence of a positive treatment effect.

A hypothetical example of the use of the ABA design is the following. A patient with limited speech output had the characteristics of a good candidate for Melodic Intonation Therapy. Once a week for 3 weeks BDAE conversational and narrative speech samples were obtained and rated. No improvement was noted. The patient then entered a course of MIT administered five times per week for 3 weeks. At the end of each week the speech samples again were obtained and rated, and improvement was noted with each retesting during the B or treatment phase. During the subsequent 3 weeks, treatment was withheld and testing showed that few changes occurred during this period. The overall pattern of test scores allowed concluding that the improvements that occurred during "the ABA study" were the result of the treatment.

Of course, some of the same issues that were raised by the multiple baseline study described previously can be restated here. First, it is not unusual for a successful course of treatment to deblock language performance, so that the patient continues to make progress after a successful course of treatment has ceased; in fact, this is a desirable consequence of treatment. Second, it may be that some other form of treatment would have been as effective as or more effective than MIT. To explore this possibility, one might choose to employ the alternating treatment design, described next.

3. **Alternating treatment design.** Sometimes two treatment approaches appear to have equal merit for a particular patient. In such cases, the clinician may choose to test the relative merits of each approach by using an alternating treatment design. For example, to compare the effectiveness of TAP with other approaches to improving confrontation naming in patients with verbal perseveration, five sessions of TAP were alternated with five sessions of another treatment suggested by the patient's profile of assets and deficits. The BDAE Confrontation Naming sub-

test was administered before treatment and then after each five-session phase to measure the generalization of treatment effects. As patients who displayed the characteristics of good candidacy for TAP were admitted to the aphasia unit, the first patient received TAP first, the second patient received the alternative treatment first, and so on. Of course, with this design it is possible that the effects achieved with one treatment may generalize to performance during the alternative treatment. But if changes occur with only one of the treatments, one can conclude that it has particular merits.

The discussion next turns to a means of measuring changes in narrative skills in patients undergoing spontaneous recovery or treatment.

II. Communicative Effectiveness Profile

The Communicative Effectiveness Profile (CEP) was developed by Menn, Helm-Estabrooks, and Ramsberger (unpublished manuscript) as an approach to analyzing BDAE "Cookie Theft" picture descriptions or other narratives. The CEP is composed of two major indices: the Index of Lexical Efficiency, which measures the ratio of informative words to total words produced, and the Index of Grammatical Support, which measures the grammaticality of the phrases that contain these informative words. This system allows a clinician to determine the extent to which a patient may display **emptiness of speech** or **agrammatic speech**. These measures may be augmented with a count of the number of **neutral probes** (e.g., "How about over here?") that the examiner had to use to obtain a more complete speech sample from the patient. Information extracted by **non-neutral probes** (e.g., "What is the mother doing?") is excluded from the analysis because the patient's task is to describe the picture in such a way that someone not familiar with its contents would have a good sense of what it depicts.

A. CEP Procedure

First, the target picture is shown to the patient, who is told "Describe everything you see going on here. Try to use full sentences." If an incomplete description is elicited, neutral probes may be used (e.g., "What about over here?"). The verbal description is tape-recorded and later transcribed and analyzed according to the following measures:

1. **Total number of words.** This is the total number of words that the patient has produced in response to the request to provide a narrative description of a pictured scene. Responses to "leading" (non-neutral) probes such as "What is *she* doing?" are excluded from the count, along with hesitation noises and interjects ("um," "er," "hm") and fragments identified as false starts on a word that eventually is produced. Fragments that seem to be identifiable as broken-off words are counted, however. Also count incorrect words, repetitions, self-corrections, jargon words, irrelevant statements, digressions, frame statements (e.g., "Now let's see here . . ."), comments (e.g., "This is a bad picture"), and so forth.

2. **Number of correct content units.** This is the number of discrete units or new bits of information supplied by the patient counting only the ones that describe correct elements of the pictures, such as "the girl," "is reaching," and "for a cookie." Only the best mention of a content unit is counted. Clinical experience shows normal controls produce an average of 18 content units, with a range of 13 to 24.

3. **Number of correct words in content units.** This is the total number of correct words that are contained within each correct content unit. Each content unit, of course, contains at least one correct word, but it may contain quite a few others as well. For example, in a unit like "I suppose he must be their mother," there are six correct words and one incorrect *(he)*, which is excluded from the count of correct words.

4. **Number of correct bound/contracted grammatical morphemes (endings) in content units.** This is the number of correct grammatical endings (plural, past, possessive -*'s*, progressing -*ing*, etc.) that the patient has used on correct words in content units. Contracted grammatical elements like the negative -*n't* and the verb forms -*'s* (as in *he's*), -*'re* (as in *they're*), and -*'ll* (as in *he'll*) are considered as endings for this purpose. Incorrect endings and endings on incorrect words or on neologisms are ignored.

Using these four numbers (total number of words, number of correct content units, number of correct words in content units, and number of correct bound/contracted grammatical morphemes in content units), proceed to compute the two indices of communicative effectiveness: the Index of Lexical Efficiency and the Index of Grammatical Support.

B. Index of Lexical Efficiency

The Index of Lexical Efficiency (ILE) is a ratio: the total number of words in the narrative response divided by the number of content units produced. The average number of words used per content unit by normal speakers is about 3.6 (range = 2.6–4.2). Aphasia patients, of course, often produce many words that are useless to the listener and that may not be part of any content unit at all. For patients with severe Wernicke's aphasia, the ILE may be over 100; that is, the patient may have produced over 100 words but said only one (e.g., *water*) that was intelligible and relevant to the picture.

C. Index of Grammatical Support

The Index of Grammatical Support (IGS) indicates the average number of "supporting words" and grammatical morphemes in each content unit. This index is computed by adding the total number of correct words in content units to the number of correct endings attached to these words and then dividing by the number of content units. The normal group produces an average of 3.5 words + endings per content unit (range = 1.8–4.7). A patient with severe Broca's aphasia who produces only endless, informative, content words (e.g., "Boy. Cookie. Water. Floor.") could have the lowest possible IGS, which is 1.0.

III. CEP Analyses of Picture Descriptions

For illustration purposes, the following examples will demonstrate the use of the Communicative Effectiveness Profile for analyzing BDAE "Cookie Theft" picture descriptions. These were obtained from one normal speaker and three aphasia patients representing a variety of aphasia classifications.

A. Normal, High School Graduate (Control Subject)

"A mother an' two kids in the kitchen. The mother is washin' dishes. The water is running in the sink. The two kids, the boy and a girl . . . . The boy is on a stool; the stool is falling. The girl is reaching for the cookies that the boy was going to get. The sink is running over. The mother is standing washing the dishes; the water's running on the floor. The stool is falling. A cup . . . two cups an' a dish in the mother's hand. The mother's standing up in the water."

Number of words: 92   **Number of probes:** 0

Content units (C.U.)	Words in C.U.	Endings in C.U.
A <u>mother</u>	2	
an' <u>two</u>	2	
<u>kids</u>	1	<u>-s</u>
in the <u>kitchen</u>	3	
(The mother) is <u>washin'</u>	4	<u>-in'</u>
<u>dishes</u>	1	<u>-s</u>
The <u>water</u>	2	
is <u>running</u>	2	<u>-ing</u>
in the <u>sink</u>	3	
(The two kids) the <u>boy</u>	5	<u>-s</u>
and a <u>girl</u>	3	
The boy is on a <u>stool</u>	6	
(the stool) is <u>falling</u>	4	<u>-ing</u>
(The girl) is <u>reaching</u>	4	<u>-ing</u>
for the <u>cookies</u>	3	<u>-s</u>
(that the boy) was <u>going to get</u>	7	<u>-ing</u>
(The sink) is running <u>over</u>	5	<u>-ing</u>
the <u>water's</u>	2	<u>-s</u>
(running) on the <u>floor</u>	4	<u>-ing</u>
<u>two</u>	1	
<u>cups</u>	1	<u>-s</u>
an' a <u>dish</u>	3	
(in the mother's) <u>hand</u>	4	<u>-'s</u>
(The mother's) <u>standing up</u> (in the water)	7	<u>-'s</u>, <u>-ing</u>
Totals: 24	79	16

Index of Lexical Efficiency: 92/24 = 3.8

Index of Grammatical Support: (79 + 16)/24 = 95/24 = 3.9

B. Broca's Aphasia

"Water. The girl down. Washing the dishes. She got . . . cookies. Fall down. He got cookies."

Number of words: 15   **Number of probes:** 0

Content units (C.U.)	Words in C.U.	Endings in C.U.
water	1	
the girl	2	
washing	1	-ing
the dishes	2	-es
Fall down	2	
He got cookies	3	-es

Totals: 6	11	3

Index of Lexical Efficiency: 15/6 = 2.5

Index of Grammatical Support: (11+3)/6 = 14/6 = 2.3

C. Wernicke's Aphasia

"All right, well there is a doll, there's a . . . here by the deed, the dilly's chilly, whatever it is. And the little voy and be and the trotty, it, it fell and the fall, and the fall, he fall down, and he's falling down on the crowd. And the water is all rinked out. Off the pipe for the end. And she, and she . . . doing the waycle. Clearing away. I'm getting all malled. And he's getting all retout and she skidded on the dill, the riddy."

Number of words: 86   **Number of probes:** 0

Content units (C.U.)	Words in C.U.	Endings in C.U.
and he's falling down	4	-'s, -ing
and the water	3	

Totals: 2	7	2

Index of Lexical Efficiency: 86/2 = 43

Index of Grammatical Support: (7+2)/2 = 9/2 = 4.5

D. Subcortical Aphasia: Posterior Capsular/Putaminal

"It's a girl . . . a short girl with long hair. He's a tenti service. The boy is scooting the jar of cookies. He's losting the bowl. The chicken, the mother . . . dishes. The fauces it off. The faucet is on. She's got the three hospital lips."

Number of words: 44   **Number of probes:** 0

Content units (C.U.)	Words in C.U.	Endings in C.U.
It's a <u>girl</u>	3	<u>-'s</u>
with <u>long hair</u>	3	
The <u>boy</u>	2	
the <u>jar</u>	2	
of <u>cookies</u>	2	<u>-es</u>
the <u>mother</u>	2	
<u>dishes</u>	1	<u>-es</u>
The <u>faucet</u>	2	
<u>is on</u>	2	

Totals: 9   19   3

Index of Grammatical Efficiency: $44/9 = 4.5$

Index of Grammatical Support: $(19+3)/9 = 22/9 = 2.4$

(*Note: Long* and *hair* are both correct informative words, so one might choose to count them as forming two units; on the other hand, most people have hair, so the separate informational value of *hair* is very low.)

IV. Using the CEP to Measure Treatment Effects

The Communicative Effectiveness Profile is a useful tool in measuring the effects of treatment. In the following case, for example, the clinician obtained "Cookie Theft" picture description samples before and after a course of treatment with the Helm Elicited Language Program for Syntax Stimulation (HELPSS; see chapter 16). The patient was a 55-year-old man with Broca's aphasia who was seen at 6.6 years post onset for treatment of agrammatism. He completed the HELPSS program in 40 hours.

A. Pre-HELPSS

"Stool . . . ah eh . . . cookies . . . eh ah . . . was . . . and ah see . . . ah . . . see . . . a bar . . . on a stool."

Number of words: 11	**Number of probes:** 0	
Content units (C.U.)	Words in C.U.	Endings in C.U.
cookies	1	-s
on a stool	3	

Totals:	2	4	1

Index of Lexical Efficiency: 11/2 = 5.5

Index of Grammatical Support: (4+1)/2 = 5/2 = 2.5

B. Post-HELPSS

"Water spills . . . . Turn it off . . . . Cookie jar and . . . ah . . . he want to give her that thing. Oh boy . . . a fall . . . fall. Sink is full. Washing the dishes."

Number of words: 26	**Number of probes:** 0	
Content units (C.U.)	Words in C.U.	Endings in C.U.
Water	1	
spills	1	-s
turn it off	3	
cookie jar	2	
he want to give her that thing	7	
a fall	2	
sink	1	
is full	2	
washing	1	-ing
the dishes	2	-s

Totals:	10	22	3

Index of Lexical Efficiency: 26/10 = 2.7

Index of Grammatical Support: (22+3)/10 = 25/10 = 2.5

By comparing pre- and post-therapy CEPs, one can see that the HELPSS program was most effective in increasing (from 2 to 10 content units) the amount of substantive information this patient could produce in a narrative description. Because therapy was instituted at 6.6 years post onset, one can attribute the significant changes in information scores to treatment rather than to spontaneous recovery. But it may be that some treatment other than HELPSS could have been as effective. To determine the relative merits of HELPSS, the clinician should have employed an alternating treatment, single-subject design such as that described previously.

References and Suggested Readings

Easterbrooks, A., Brown, B.B., & Perera, K. (1982). A comparison of the speech of adult aphasic subjects in spontaneous and structured interactions. *British Journal of Disorders of Communication, 17*(3), 93–107.

Fitzpatrick, P., Glosser, & Helm-Estabrooks, N. (1988, October). *Long-term recovery of linguistic and non-linguistic function in aphasia.* Paper presented at the annual meeting of the Academy of Aphasia, Montreal.

Goodglass, H., & Kaplan, E. (1984). *Aphasia and related disorders.* Philadelphia: Lea & Febiger.

Holland, A.L. (1980). *Communicative Abilities in Daily Living.* Austin, TX: PRO-ED.

Holland, A.L. (1982). Observing functional communication in aphasic adults. *Journal of Speech and Hearing Disorders, 17,* 50–56.

Kearns, K.P. (1986). Flexibility of single-subject experimental designs. Part II: Design selection and arrangement of experimental phases. *Journal of Speech and Hearing Disorders, 51,* 204–214.

McReynolds, L.V., & Thompson, C.K. (1986). Flexibility of single-subject experimental designs. Part I: Review of the basics of single-subject designs. *Journal of Speech and Hearing Disorders, 51,* 194–203.

Naeser, M., & Helm-Estabrooks, N. (1985). CT scan lesion localization and response to Melodic Intonation Therapy with nonfluent aphasia cases. *Cortex, 21,* 203–223.

Rosenbek, J., LaPointe, L., & Wertz, R. (1989). *Aphasia: A clinical approach.* Austin, TX: PRO-ED.

Shewan, C.M. (1986). The history and efficacy of aphasia treatment. In R. Chapey (Ed.), *Language intervention strategies in adult aphasia* (2nd ed., pp. 28–43). Baltimore: Williams & Wilkins.

Section Four
Specific
Therapy Programs

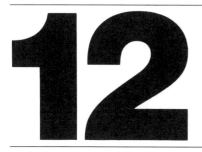

Visual Action Therapy

A significant number of patients referred for early aphasia rehabilitation have global aphasia. In linguistic terms, global aphasia is the inability to produce and understand spoken and written language. In addition to these deficits, the globally aphasic individual may have severe apraxia, which interferes with nonverbal means of expression such as gesturing and drawing. Such patients, then, show poor ability to communicate through any modality. Unfortunately, attempts to treat global aphasia with traditional language-based approaches were shown to be largely ineffective. This observation led some aphasiologists to believe that globally aphasic patients suffer a loss of the underlying linguistic rules and cognitive operations needed for language.

In the 1970s psychologists began to explore the issue of language competency in global aphasia through the use of alternate symbol systems. One of these landmark studies was undertaken by Gardner, Zurif, Berry, and Baker (1976). These researchers used a **visual communication (VIC) system** consisting of real objects and a series of index cards containing simple, arbitrary, or representational drawings denoting meaningful units. Patients were required to carry out operations such as following commands, answering questions, and describing events by manipulating the objects and cards. Based on the patients' performance with these tasks, the investigators concluded that global patients do retain a rich conceptual system and at least some of the cognitive operations necessary for natural language. In addition, five of the eight VIC patients showed significant gains on a test of auditory comprehension, despite the fact that VIC was carried out in silence.

A. The Visual Action Therapy Approach

The VIC findings encouraged Helm and Benson (1978) to explore the use of a nonvocal, visual/gestural approach to the rehabilitation of globally aphasic patients. This research led to the development of a method called Visual Action Therapy (VAT), which trained severely aphasic patients to represent hidden items with hand/arm gestures. The effect of VAT on eight globally aphasic patients was reported in Helm-Estabrooks, Fitzpatrick, and Barresi (1982). All eight had failed to respond to traditional language approaches, but with VAT, highly significant changes occurred on the *Porch Index of Communicative Ability* (PICA; Porch, 1981) subtests of auditory comprehension and pantomime. No significant changes occurred on tests of verbal expression, however, but this might have been due to the fact that the patients continued to demonstrate marked bucco/facial apraxia. The VAT method subsequently was expanded to include a program for bucco/facial apraxia, in which all representational gestures involve the mouth/face. Six patients treated with bucco/facial VAT showed significant improvement in PICA verbal repetition scores as well as in pantomime, auditory comprehension, reading comprehension, and graphic copy (Ramsberger & Helm-Estabrooks, 1988).

A final modification emerged from an item-difficulty study (Helm-Estabrooks, Ramsberger, Brownell, & Albert, 1985) that arose from the observation that it was relatively easier to train patients to gesturally represent objects involving proximal movements than distal movements (see chapter 9 for definitions). Training data from 12 globally aphasic, apraxic patients confirmed that proximal gestures (e.g., sawing) were significantly easier to train than distal gestures (e.g., turning a screwdriver). The results of this study led to the creation of Proximal Limb Visual Action Therapy and Distal Limb Visual Action Therapy.

All three VAT programs use real objects, line drawings of these objects, and pictures of a simple figure using the objects (see examples in Fig. 12.1). Each program consists of hierarchically ordered steps and levels that move the patient along a performance continuum from the basic task of matching pictures and objects to the communicative task of representing hidden items with self-initiated gestures. Score sheets are used to document performance carefully and to determine movement from one step or level to the next. Finally, dependent test variables are used to measure the overall effectiveness of the programs.

B. Candidacy for Visual Action Therapy

Candidacy studies on Visual Action Therapy, including that of Biber, Helm-Estabrooks, Fitzpatrick, and Wysocki (1983), have allowed the identification of many of the features that suggest good or poor response to VAT. The good candidate for VAT will

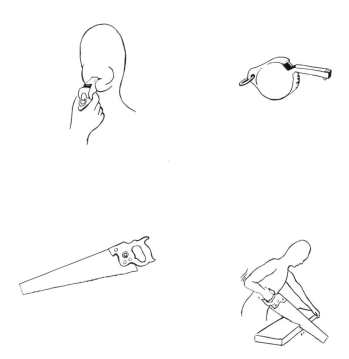

FIG. 12.1. Examples of Visual Action Therapy picture stimuli

have not only the ability to complete the steps and levels of the program but will show improvement on some dependent measure of communication as a result of this treatment.

Good candidates for limb VAT will have all of the following characteristics:

Pre-treatment characteristics of good limb VAT candidates:

1. **Etiology:** unilateral, left-hemisphere stroke(s).

2. **Lesion(s):** confined to the left cerebral hemisphere but may include or undercut most of the primary language zones.

3. **Aphasia type:** global or near global aphasia with severely restricted expression and comprehension of spoken and written language.

4. **Praxis:** moderate to severe intransitive and transitive limb apraxia.

5. **Psychological features:** alert, oriented, and cooperative with good attention span.

Good candidates for bucco/facial VAT will have all of the following characteristics:

Pre-treatment characteristics of good bucco/facial VAT candidates:

1. **Etiology:** unilateral, left-hemisphere stroke.

2. **Lesion:** involves or undercuts the anterior language areas of the left cerebral hemisphere.

3. **Aphasia type:** severely restricted verbal output despite moderately preserved or recovered auditory skills.

4. **Praxis:** moderate to severe bucco/facial apraxia despite moderately preserved or recovered limb praxis.

5. **Psychological features:** cooperative and well motivated with good attention span.

In addition to the preceding characteristics, candidates for either limb or bucco/facial VAT should show at least moderate ability to perform the following neuropsychological tests:

Neuropsychological tasks for determining VAT candidacy:

1. **Delayed recognition of designs:** Wechsler Memory Scale

2. **Stick designs from memory:** BDAE "Parietal Lobe" Battery

3. **Object assembly:** WAIS-R Performance Scale

4. **Drawings to command and copy:** BDAE "Parietal Lobe" Battery

5. **Symbol discrimination:** BDAE

C. **Preparing for a Visual Action Therapy Session**

For each of the three VAT programs (proximal limb, distal limb, and bucco/facial), the clinician must obtain the following items: seven real objects, seven shaded line drawings of these items, and seven pictures of a simple figure using these items ("action" pictures). In addition to the VAT objects, some contextual props are required (e.g., a screw in a block of wood for use with the screwdriver). Score sheets are prepared for recording trial-by-trial performance and for determining progress along the task continuum. VAT sessions last approximately 30 minutes, and inpatients may be seen twice a day to accelerate progress through the program.

1. **Visual Action Therapy objects**

    a. **Proximal limb VAT:** American flag, meat grinder, paint stick, gavel, paint roller, saw, and iron.

    b. **Distal limb VAT:** screwdriver, pencil sharpener, teaspoon, telegraph key, picture paintbrush, dial telephone, and tea bag.

    c. **Bucco/facial VAT:** whistle, artificial carnation, lollipop, drinking straw, Chapstick, razor, and kaleidoscope.

2. **Contextual props**

    a. **Proximal limb VAT:** empty gallon paint can (for stirring with paint stick) and small length of wood (for sawing).

    b. **Distal limb VAT:** block of wood containing a large screw (for turning with screwdriver), coffee mug (for stirring with teaspoon), and paint-by-number outline of picture (for painting with small paint brush).

    c. **Bucco/facial VAT:** soft drink bottle (for drinking through straw) and floral essence or perfume (to scent artificial carnation).

None of the VAT objects are toys; they are real objects, obtained from hardware or variety stores (or attics and cellars). For example, a broken iron will do, and the dial section of the telephone is sufficient. One might find a gavel at a trophy store and a telegraph key at Radio Shack. The paint-by-number picture can be photocopied for multiple trials or patients.

D. **The Scoring Procedure**

Not all the steps of Visual Action Therapy can be scored. Steps 3, 5, and 8 are for demonstration purposes only, so that the patient has only to attend to the clinician's activities (the nonscorable steps are identified by the word *demonstration*). The scoring system used in all three VAT programs is simple. One

(1) point is given for a fully correct performance without great hesitation or groping, one half (.5) point is given for a greatly delayed or self-corrected performance, and a score of zero (0) is assigned to all other attempts. (At the same time, the clinician should note the *nature* of the incorrect responses.) Because each program has seven objects, a perfect score is 7.0. In order to move from one step to the next, the patient must earn an overall score of 6.5, allowing for one self-correction. If multiple trials are required for a particular step, then the average score for three consecutive trials must be higher than the average score for the three previous trials, or the clinician must consider whether the program is appropriate for the patient. Before discontinuing the program, however, modifications may be made on the basis of the patient's errors.

In addition to scoring the performances, the clinician records **paramimias** (substitution of one gesture for another) and **perseverations** with margin notes. This process allows one to modify the order of item presentation to maximize the patient's performance. For example, if the patient continues to produce the gesture for ironing whenever the saw is presented after the iron (a perseverative response), then the saw should not be offered immediately after the iron in the first stages of training. In the case of a consistent paramimia, such as the substitution of the gesture for telephone dial whenever the telegraph key is presented, the clinician may want to substitute another distal object for the key.

E. VAT Steps and Levels

Each of the three programs in Visual Action Therapy has three levels. The first level employs real objects as well as pictures of the object and the action pictures. Level I consists of nine steps (note that step 1 is actually made up of four substeps), descriptions of which follow:

1. **Matching pictures and objects.** The goal of this step is to assure that the patient has the visuospatial and symbolic skills necessary for matching objects with line drawings of these objects. This is accomplished through four hierarchically ordered substeps. *Note:* If the patient is not able to complete the first of these substeps accurately, a trial of tracing, in which the clinician and then the patient traces a few of the objects, may help. The patient later places the objects on the appropriate outline. This maneuver is some-

times successful in establishing "set" for step 1. If the patient cannot complete step 1 even with a trial of tracing, then VAT probably is not appropriate and another treatment approach should be explored.

a. **Placing objects on pictures.** Sitting across from the patient, place all seven line drawings of the objects on the table in random order. Hand each object (without props) to the patient (in another random order) and indicate silently that he or she is to lay the object on its pictorial representation. Because the objects are not removed until all seven are in place, the task becomes easier and easier as the choices narrow from seven to six to five and so on. When the patient has achieved a score of 6.5 (one delay only) or better, introduce step b.

b. **Placing pictures on objects.** Arrange all seven objects randomly before the patient and hand the pictures to him or her in a different random order. Silently encourage the patient to lay the pictures on the objects they represent. As in step 1a, this task becomes easier as the choices narrow. When the patient has earned a score of 6.5 (one delay) or better, begin step c.

c. **Pointing to objects.** Collect the pictures and rearrange the objects. Then hold up the pictures one at a time and nonverbally indicate that the patient must *point to* (not pick up) the object represented by the picture. *Note:* Some severely apraxic patients cannot isolate and extend the nonhemiplegic index finger for pointing. In these cases, place a red dot (sticker) on the objects and pictures and model the pointing behavior by helping the patient to extend only his or her index finger and touch the dot. In the severest cases, wrap tape around the finger, removing it later when the behavior becomes more entrenched. Similarly, the red dots are removed and the patient completes this step without these aids before progressing to step d.

d. **Pointing to pictures.** Arrange all seven cards before the patient. Then hold up the objects one by one and indicate that the patient should *point to* (not pick up) the object associated with each picture. Red dots may be placed on the objects to encourage pointing, but if the patient has successfully completed step 1c, he or she should have the praxic skills necessary for pointing. When the patient earns an overall score of 6.5 on any one trial of this step, introduce step 2.

2. **Object use training.** The goal of this step is to assure that the patient has the necessary praxis skills for appropriate manipulation of real objects. To demonstrate these skills, the patient must pick and position the item and carry out its associated action. Present each object (and any contextual prop) separately and demonstrate its use for the patient (e.g., saw the wood). Then place (do not hand) the object on the table in front of the patient and encourage him or her to pick it up and demonstrate its use. This may require some modeling and shaping, but the patient must be able to manipulate the object properly without assistance in order to receive credit. Once the 6.5 criterion has been reached, introduce step 3.

3. **Action picture demonstration.** The goal of this nonscorable step is for the patient to appreciate that each action picture represents a "command" to pick up the real object and carry out the associated action. Randomly choose an object and the action picture of the figure manipulating that object. Place the object in front of the patient and the corresponding action picture slightly to the patient's left. Point to the picture and then pick up the object and demonstrate its use. Do this for each of the action picture/object combinations.

4. **Following action picture commands.** The goal of this step is for the patient to choose the correct object from the random array of seven and manipulate it appropriately when shown a corresponding action picture. Place all seven objects with props in front of (but slightly away from) the patient. Hold up an action picture and show it to the patient until he or she has correctly selected and manipulated the corresponding object. If modeling or shaping is required or if a score of less than 6.5 is earned, give subsequent trials of this step until that criterion for advancement to step 5 is achieved.

5. **Pantomimed gesture demonstration.** The goal of this nonscorable step is to demonstrate to the patient that pantomimed gestures can "stand for" or represent objects. Place each object (slightly away from the patient and without

contextual props) on the table and produce the gesture that best represents the object. Proceed slowly so that the patient can cognitively link the gestures with the objects.

Note: At this point all contextual props are eliminated.

6. **Pantomimed gesture recognition.** In this step the patient must show that he or she associates pantomimed gestures with the objects they represent. Place all seven objects in a random order on the table and produce a pantomimed gesture representing one of the objects. Silently encourage the patient to locate/point to the corresponding object. When a score of 6.5 or 7.0 has been earned, introduce step 7.

7. **Pantomimed gesture production.** The goal of this step is to train the patient to produce appropriate, representational gestures for each of the seven objects. One by one, show each of the seven objects to the patient, encouraging him or her to produce a correct, representational gesture without touching the object. This may require some modeling and imitation. In extreme cases, the patient may need to manipulate the actual object; while slowly withdrawing it, encourage the patient to continue the gesture without the object. In order to receive full credit, the patient must produce a correct, pantomimed gesture upon looking at the object. Half credit may be earned for a self-corrected or delayed performance. Introduce step 8 only when the patient has earned an overall score of 6.5 or better.

8. **Representation of hidden objects demonstration.** The goal of this step is for the patient to understand that representational gestures can "stand for" hidden objects; that is, that a message can convey a concept not visually present. Choose two of the objects and place them on the table one at a time while producing a representational gesture for each. Then hide the two objects under a box. Remove one object and produce a gesture to represent the remaining hidden item. In this manner, each object takes its turn remaining under the box to be represented with a gesture. Because this is merely a demonstration, the patient earns no credit. Step 9 is introduced once the demonstration is complete.

9. **Production of gestures for hidden objects.** The goal of this final step of Level I is for the patient to gesturally

represent hidden objects; that is, to convey a message about something that cannot be seen. Place two randomly selected objects on the table and encourage the patient to produce gestures for each. Hide the objects then under a box. After about 6 seconds, remove one object and indicate that the patient should produce a gesture for the one that remains hidden. Do this for all possible pairs until each of the seven objects has remained hidden for purposes of gestural representation. When the patient earns a score of 6.5 or better for this step, introduce Level II at step 5.

In VAT Level II, no real objects are employed; instead, the action pictures are substituted for the objects beginning with step 5. Only steps 6, 7, and 9 are scorable, however, so this level is relatively brief. In VAT Level III, only the pictures of the objects are employed. As in Level II, this final level also begins with step 5. Upon completion of Level III of proximal limb VAT, distal limb VAT is introduced at Level I, step 1. Following the two limb VAT programs, the patient with bucco/facial apraxia should receive a course of bucco/facial VAT. The latter uses the same levels and steps as the limb VAT programs.

F. Measuring Response to Visual Action Therapy

The goal of limb VAT is to reduce apraxia and improve the patient's ability to use symbolic gestures as a means of communication. The goal of bucco/facial VAT is to reduce bucco/facial apraxia and improve verbal expression. To measure the effectiveness of the programs in attaining these goals, it is necessary to select one or more clinical tools that will serve as the dependent variable. It is assumed that some test of limb and bucco/facial apraxia will be administered previous to initiating the programs; these results, then, can serve as one measure of response to VAT treatment. Borod, Fitzpatrick, Helm-Estabrooks, and Goodglass (1988) compared scores earned by patients on the apraxia test described in chapter 9 with ratings earned on a nonvocal communication scale (NCS) and found the two measures highly correlated. In other words, the results of the apraxia test were predictive of how well the patient used gestures to communicate in his or her natural environment. The clinical implication of this finding is that the clinician may choose either tool (apraxia test or NCS) as a measure of the patient's gestural communication skills.

In the previously cited group study of limb VAT (Helm-Estabrooks, Fitzpatrick, & Barresi, 1982) the *Porch Index of Communicative Ability* was administered before and after treatment, revealing that the pantomime subtests II and III and the auditory comprehension subtests VI and X were particularly sensitive to positive changes in performance with VAT treatment. Further, a study of bucco/facial VAT (Ramsberger & Helm-Estabrooks, 1988) showed that PICA subtest XII (Repetition of Nouns) was sensitive to changes in verbalization. Thus, these particular PICA subtests are recommended as measures of performances changes with VAT treatment.

References and Suggested Readings

Biber, C., Helm-Estabrooks, N., Fitzpatrick, P., & Wysocki, D. (1983, October). *Predicting responses to an aphasia treatment program with neuropsychological test results.* Paper presented at the annual meeting of the Academy of Aphasia, Minneapolis.

Borod, J., Fitzpatrick, P., Helm-Estabrooks, N., & Goodglass, H. (1989). The relationship between limb apraxia and the spontaneous use of communicative gesture in aphasia. *Brain and Cognition, 10,* 121–131.

Gardner, H., Zurif, E., Berry, T., & Baker, E. (1976). Visual communication in aphasia. *Neuropsychologia, 14,* 275–292.

Helm, N.A., & Benson, D.F. (1978, October). *Visual Action Therapy for global aphasia.* Paper presented at the annual meeting of the Academy of Aphasia, Chicago.

Helm-Estabrooks, N., & Emery, P. (1988). Nonvocal approaches to aphasia rehabilitation. In F. Rose, R. Whurr, & M. Wyke (Eds.), *Aphasia* (pp. 473–487). London: Whurr Publishers.

Helm-Estabrooks, N., Fitzpatrick, P., & Barresi, B. (1982). Visual Action Therapy for global aphasia. *Journal of Speech and Hearing Disorders, 44,* 385–389.

Helm-Estabrooks, N., Ramsberger, G., Brownell, H., & Albert, M. (1989). Distal versus proximal movement in limb apraxia [Abstract]. *Journal of Clinical and Experimental Neuropsychology, 7,* 608.

Porch, B.E. (1981). *Porch Index of Communicative Ability.* Palo Alto, CA: Consulting Psychologists Press.

Ramsberger, G., & Helm-Estabrooks, N. (1988). Visual Action Therapy for bucco-facial apraxia. In *Clinical Aphasiology Conference Proceedings.* Austin, TX: PRO-ED.

13 "Back to the Drawing Board"

Some severely aphasic patients remain unable to communicate verbally despite intensive speech therapy. In some cases this failure to regain speech may be attributed to the location and extent of the brain lesion in the medial subcallosal fasciculus and other white-matter pathways (Naeser, Palumbo, Helm-Estabrooks, Stiassney-Eder, & Albert, 1989). For such individuals a nonlinguistic system, such as drawing, may serve as a means of communication. For example, de Ajuriaguerra and Hécaen (1950) described a patient with "marked jargon aphasia" who spontaneously resorted to drawing events such as the collision of his bicycle and a horse-drawn vehicle. Similarly, a patient who was unable to tell us where he was from drew a picture that allowed us to guess correctly "the state of Maine" (see Fig 13.1).

Despite the fact that many aphasic patients have the capacity for communicating a message through drawing, few drawing programs for aphasia rehabilitation have been described. One exception is found in a 1974 study by Hatfield and Zangwill, who trained one nonfluent patient to draw pictures that conveyed short stories narrated to him, scenes acted out by the clinician, and events occurring in his own life. Although this patient had no particular premorbid artistic skills, his drawings

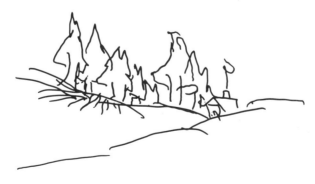

FIG. 13.1. Spontaneous drawing from an aphasic patient

189

indicated that his ideational processes were relatively intact despite his verbal deficits.

Another such case study (de Lorant & van Eeckhout, 1980) described a French patient called Sabadel who was a graphic illustrator before the onset of right hemiplegia and global aphasia. With encouragement, Sabadel began to draw simple objects and then complete agent, action, and object concepts using his nonpreferred left hand. Eventually, he was able to illustrate a book that described his recovery process (Pillon, Signoret, van Eeckhout, & Lhermitte, 1980).

One of the first group treatment studies to use a drawing program was conducted by Lyon and Sims (1986). Five patients with right hemiplegia and severely restricted verbal expression were trained to draw personally salient themes or "happenings" (e.g., the patient sitting in his living room reading the newspaper). Before and after treatment, the subjects were asked to convey to naive interactants 40 untrained concepts under two test conditions: (a) verbal and/or gestural description of the messages, and (b) graphic illustration of the messages to the interactants through drawing. Before treatment, subjects were better able to convey concepts through drawing than they were through verbal and/or gestural descriptions. After treatment the advantage of the drawing condition was even greater. A description of some of the training strategies used by Lyon and Sims can be found in Lyon and Helm-Estabrooks (1987).

In 1987 Morgan and Helm-Estabrooks described a drawing program used with two severely aphasic patients who had shown minimal response to various speech therapies. As a pretest the patients were required to depict daily mishaps enacted by a clinician (e.g., dropping a handful of papers). They then entered the training program, which required them first to draw cartoons to visual memory, then to refine them through copy, and finally to execute them again to memory. (See Fig. 13.2 for an example of a one-panel cartoon drawn from memory before and after the copy condition.) Once the patients were able to depict themes and important details of the cartoons to memory, the pretest was readministered. These pre- and post-treatment test drawings (see Fig. 13.3 for an example) then were given to naive judges, who were better able to identify the crucial elements in the post-treatment drawings. Both patients in this study went on to use drawing as a means of communication at home and in their aphasia group meetings. Fig. 13.4 shows an example of a communicative drawing produced in response to the question "What did you do over the weekend?"

PT. B PRE- AND POST-TREATMENT CARTOON REPRODUCTIONS.

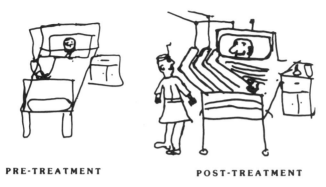

PRE-TREATMENT   POST-TREATMENT

FIG. 13.2. Cartoon drawn from memory before and after copy condition

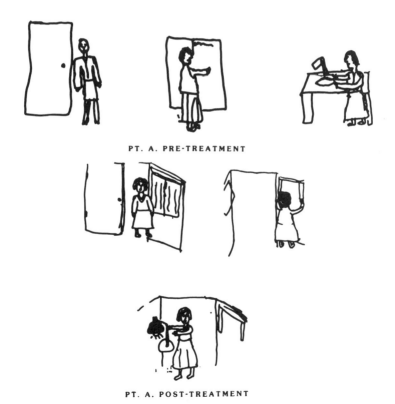

PT. A. PRE-TREATMENT

PT. A. POST-TREATMENT

FIG. 13.3. Pre- and post-treatment drawings of a three-part enacted scene ("Woman entering dark room, opening drapes, and turning on light")

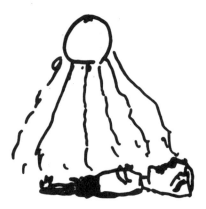

FIG. 13.4. Spontaneous drawing post therapy

In all of the preceding studies, the patients have been severely non-fluent. In 1989, however, Young and Helm-Estabrooks reported that both fluent and nonfluent aphasic patients could draw items they were never able to name correctly. Equally important was the finding that patients often were able to verbalize the correct response during the act of drawing. The results of this study suggest that a drawing program may stimulate verbal communication. Similarly, drawing may deblock written expression in some patients. In any case, a drawing program has its own intrinsic value for patients who are unable to communicate through speech or writing. For this reason, the program Morgan and Helm-Estabrooks (1987) called "Back to the Drawing Board" is described next.

A. The "Back to the Drawing Board" Program

"Back to the Drawing Board" (BDB) is designed to encourage aphasic individuals who are severely impaired in verbal expression to communicate feelings, needs, and events through drawing. The stimuli used in this program consist of single-, double-, and triple-panel uncaptioned cartoons. The use of cartoons is based on research evidence (Gardner, Ling, Flamm, & Silverman, 1975) that even severely aphasic patients may appreciate visual humor in the form of cartoons. Furthermore, the emotional value of the stimuli (e.g., humor or anger) often enhances the performance of aphasic patients. Finally, the simple line-drawing style of cartoons is relatively easy to copy.

The within-treatment goal of BDB is for the patient to produce an acceptable rendition of the cartoon stimuli to memory. The criterion for acceptability is that both the main theme(s) and the critical details of the cartoon are present and recognizable to a naive judge. This goal is accomplished through copy of the target stimuli with instruction and demonstration from the clinician.

The ultimate goal of the BDB program is for the patient to use drawing for everyday communication when other means of exchange are unsuccessful. To assess the patient's potential capacity for the functional use of drawing, a pre-/post-treatment drawing measure called the *Daily Mishaps Test* was developed (description follows). In addition, the clinician should ask patients, families, or caretakers to report instances of the functional use of drawing and to show copies of these drawings.

B. Candidacy for the BDB Program

Patients who are considered for the BDB program should meet all of the following criteria:

1. The patient should have a *Boston Diagnostic Aphasia Examination* (BDAE) Severity Rating of 1.0 or 1.5, indicating that, at best, communication takes place through fragmentary expression with the need for inference, questioning, and guessing by the listener.

2. Scores on the BDAE auditory comprehension subtests should be at least at the 60th percentile.

3. The man drawn for the *Boston Assessment of Severe Aphasia* (BASA) should earn a score of 2, indicating that it is immediately recognizable as a man (see Fig. 13.5).

4. The patient should be able to place three, triple-panel, uncaptioned cartoons in the proper sequence.

5. The patient should be able to point out the humorous element in six single-panel, uncaptioned cartoons.

C. Preparing for a BDB Session

After determining that a patient is a good candidate for a drawing program, the clinician next should explain the merits of such a program to him or her. The clinician then prepares or locates 12 bold-line, uncaptioned cartoon stimuli (5 single-panel, 4 double-panel, and 3 triple-panel) designed to encour-

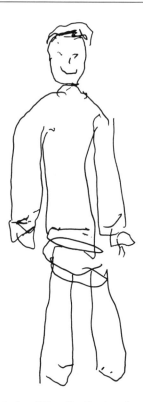

FIG. 13.5. Drawing of man rated as G2 on the *Boston Assessment of Severe Aphasia*

age the accurate portrayal of objects, people, facial expressions, actions, and single and serial events. Single-panel cartoons (such as that in Fig. 13.6) introduce the concepts of global configuration, external and internal detail, relative size, and three-dimensionality. In these one-panel cartoons the crucial details should be on the left side or in the center of the space because patients with left-brain damage often show inattention to details presented in the right hemiattentional field. The two- and three-panel cartoons should elaborate on the themes present in single panels and introduce the concepts of action, passage of time, and sequential events. Drawing stimuli are important; if the stimuli are taken from existing compilations of cartoons (found in most libraries), avoid those with a highly ornate or detailed style.

The only other materials required for the BDB program are white index cards and a felt-tip pen. For each attempt to draw a

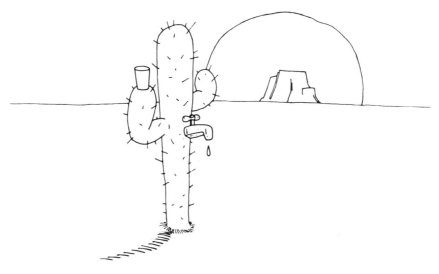

FIG. 13.6. Example of a one-panel cartoon stimulus

cartoon, give the patient the appropriate number of unlined 5″ × 5″ cards (e.g., three cards for a three-panel cartoon). Analyze the patient's attempts vis-à-vis the model drawings so that the patient's errors can be identified and corrected. By saving all drawing attempts, one can document trial-to-trial improvement.

D. The Daily Mishaps Test

An assessment tool called the *Daily Mishaps Test* (DMT), given just prior to and just after completion of the BDB program, is used to measure the effects of the program on the aphasic patient's ability to communicate through drawing. In this test, the patient observes scenes enacted by a person other than the treating clinician. Following each scene the patient is presented with either one, two, or three 5″ × 5″ cards for depicting the scene just enacted. Descriptions of the scenes follow:

1. One-part scenes

  a. A woman puts up an umbrella in which one spoke is broken and dangling.

  b. A woman leaning on a desk knocks a book on the floor.

  c. A woman pours water into a cup that has a hole in the bottom and the water leaks out.

2. Two-part scenes

   a. A woman is shuffling cards. She then loses control of them and they scatter all over the table.

   b. A woman comes into the room carrying a stack of books. She tips the stack and the top one falls to the floor.

   c. A woman turns on a fan. As the fan rotates, the papers on a desk blow around.

3. Three-part scenes

   a. A woman waters a plant on the window sill. She spills some water. She wipes up the water with paper towels.

   b. A woman begins writing on a pad of paper. The point on the pencil breaks. The woman sharpens the pencil.

   c. A woman walks into a dark room. She turns on the light. Then she opens the drapes.

E. Implementation of the BDB Program

After a pre-test with the DMT, the clinician initiates the BDB program. As in other programs, however, these steps should be modified or augmented according to the individual patient's performance. Allowances should be made for use of the non-preferred hand, but the drawings (although they may not be considered "artistic") should convey the correct message.

1. Present the patient with a one-panel, uncaptioned cartoon and let him or her study it before turning it over. Then ask the patient to draw the cartoon from memory on an unlined 5″ × 5″ card.

2. Evaluate the patient's rendition of the target cartoon.

   a. If the main theme (e.g., a man snorkeling) is recognizable and the picture contains the detail(s) critical to the scene's humor (e.g., a fishing hook is pulling the man up by the bathing suit), then present a new single-panel cartoon at step 1.

   b. If the main theme is not identifiable or if critical elements are missing or unclear, work with the patient to improve his or her performance. This may include pointing out the deficiencies, drawing elements for copy, or encouraging enlargement of crucial details. Once the patient is able to copy the target cartoon correctly, turn it over and again ask for a drawing from memory on a blank card. If the drawing is unsatisfactory, repeat this step up to three more times before eliminating the too-difficult cartoon and beginning again with a new cartoon. Whenever a target is accurately drawn from memory, introduce a new cartoon at step 1.

3. Once the patient has drawn five single-panel, uncaptioned cartoons from memory, introduce the first of the two-panel cartoons at step 1 using two bank 5″ × 5″ cards. Repeat the steps until four recognizable double-panel cartoons can be drawn from memory. At this point introduce the first of the three-panel cartoons with three blank cards for step 1. When three recognizable, triple-panel cartoons have been drawn from memory, readminister the Daily Mishaps Test.

Following the BDB program, the clinician should give the two (pre- and post-treatment) sets of DMT drawings to a naive rater, requesting that he or she try to write a description of the main theme and the details conveyed by the patient's drawings. The clinician then assesses whether the DMT target events were best conveyed by the pre- or post-BDB drawing. If the patient has improved in his or her ability to depict the DMT events through drawing, then a second, less formal phase of training is begun.

F. Post-BDB Training

Following successful completion of the cartoon program, a less structured program involving family members or caretakers is initiated. The goal of this phase of training is for the patient to successfully convey a unique message to the interactant. Because many untrained individuals do not know how best to extract information from the drawings of aphasic patients, one can train the interactant to use the questioning strategies suggested by Lyon and Sims (see Lyon & Helm-Estabrooks, 1987). These include identifying general themes (e.g., "Is it a building?"), identifying elements (e.g., "Is this a picture on the wall?"), using interactive drawing (e.g., "Is it square, like this?"), and encouraging multimodal expression (e.g., "Can you show me with a gesture?"). Model these strategies first for the family members by asking them to identify unique messages for the patient to convey to the clinician (e.g., where the patient and his wife went on Saturday), then give the patient messages to relate to the family members. Even if the patient and family members communicate successfully within this format, the better test of the effectiveness of the drawing program is the extent to which daily communication improves. It is difficult, of course, to measure this improvement, but through anecdotal information and drawings provided by patients or family members, one can try to judge the generalized effects of the training.

References and Suggested Readings

de Ajuriaguerra, J., & Hécaen, H. (1950). *Le cortex cérébral: Étude neuro-psych-pathologique* [Cerebral cortex: A neuro-psycho-pathological study]. Paris: Masson.

de Lorant, G., & van Eeckhout, P. (1980). *Sabadel: L'homme qui ne savait plus parler* [Sabadel: The man who no longer knew how to speak]. Baudiniere, France: Nouvelles Editions.

Gardner, H., Ling, P.K., Flamm, L., & Silverman, J. (1975). Comprehension and appreciation of humorous material following brain damage. *Brain, 98,* 399–412.

Hatfield, F.M., & Zangwill, O.L. (1974). Ideation in aphasia: The picture-story method. *Neuropsychologia, 12,* 389–393.

Helm-Estabrooks, N., Ramsberger, G., Morgan, A., & Nicholas, M. (1989). *Boston Assessment of Severe Aphasia.* San Antonio, TX: Special Press.

Lyon, J., & Helm-Estabrooks, N. (1987). Drawing: Its communicative significance for expressively restricted aphasic adults. *Topics in Language Disorders, 8*(1), 61–71.

Lyon, J.G., & Sims, E. (1986, June). *Drawing: Evaluation of its use as a communicative aid with aphasic and normal adults.* Paper presented at the Second International Aphasia Rehabilitation Conference, Göteborg, Sweden.

Morgan, A., & Helm-Estabrooks, N. (1987). Back to the Drawing Board: A treatment program for nonverbal aphasic patients. In R.H. Brookshire (Ed.), *Clinical Aphasiology Conference Proceedings.* Minneapolis, MN: BRK.

Naeser, M.A., Palumbo, C., Helm-Estabrooks,N., Stiassney-Eder, D., & Albert, M.L. (1989). Severe nonfluency in aphasia. *Brain, 112,* 1–38.

Pillon, B., Signoret, J.L., van Eeckhout, P., & Lhermitte, F. (1980). Le dessin chez un aphasique. Incidence possible sur le langage et sa reeducation [Drawing for the aphasic: The possible impact of language and its reeducation]. *Revue Neurologique, 136,* 699–710.

Young, S., & Helm-Estabrooks, N. (1989, October). *Drawing and responsive naming in aphasia.* Paper presented at the annual meeting of the Academy of Aphasia, Santa Fe, NM.

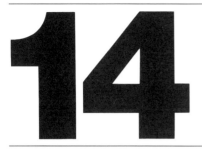

Voluntary Control of Involuntary Utterances

In 1878 Hughlings Jackson described aphasia as a disorder in the ability to use language intentionally, stating that the higher the propositional value of a task, the less the aphasic patient will be able to respond to it. He went on to observe that the more automatic, emotional, or contextual the nature of the task, the more likely that the aphasic patient would produce appropriate utterances. Thus one sees patients who cannot produce words in response to an aphasia test but subsequently say "good-bye" when leaving the examining room.

During the 100-year history of aphasia therapy, occasional aphasiologists have suggested that this dissociation of ability to produce automatic versus propositional speech may serve as a basis for rehabilitation. Huber (1944) observed that even if the words and phrases uttered automatically are incorrect, they are valuable cues to the sounds a patient is capable of producing. Similarly, Goda (1962) suggested that clinicians could use a patient's attempts at producing spontaneous speech to determine treatment vocabulary, rather than relying on prepared materials for rehabilitation.

In a 1964 study of aphasia rehabilitation, Vignolo summarized one approach to treatment as follows: "First an automatic way to elicit a correct response is found, and the response is then tentatively elicited in more and more voluntary ways" (p. 349). This echoed the words of Sheehan, who said "we [should] capitalize on involuntary speech and raise it to a voluntary level" (1946, p. 151).

It was not until 1980, however, that the concept of bringing involuntary speech utterances under voluntary control for purposes of aphasia rehabilitation was explored systematically. In that year, Helm and Barresi described a method called Voluntary Control of Involuntary Utterances (VCIU), in which oral reading was used as the first step toward propositional speech. Three patients whose intentional attempts to communicate were limited to a few stereotypic expressions such as "I don't know" and "real good" were enrolled in a course of VCIU. They ranged in time post onset from 2 months to 3 years when enrolled in

VCIU. All had shown poor verbal response to other therapies. After 3 to 6 months of VCIU, all showed significant improvement in naming-test scores and conversational skills.

A. The Voluntary Control of Involuntary Utterances Program

Voluntary Control of Involuntary Utterances, or VCIU, is an approach to improving verbal output in severely nonfluent aphasic patients whose speech is limited to the stereotypic production of a few real words. Oral reading of patient-produced utterances forms the basis of VCIU, and the sequence of tasks moves from (a) oral reading to (b) confrontation naming to (c) conversational use of these words or phrases. Thus, it progresses from a relatively automatic task to a more voluntary or propositional task. VCIU is based on the belief that virtually all aphasic patients have the ability to utter real words under some circumstance. The burden is on the clinician to identify this core involuntary vocabulary and help the patient bring it under voluntary control.

B. Candidacy for VCIU

Patients who will respond well to VCIU initially have most or all of the following characteristics:

1. **Etiology:** unilateral, left-hemisphere stroke.

2. **Lesion site:** often (but not necessarily) mainly subcortical.

3. **Speech output:** severely limited, often to a few real words used in a stereotypic manner.

4. **Reading:** can match words correctly to pictured objects and actions. Oral reading may be inconsistent, with some tendency to utter incorrect, but related, words to stimuli (e.g., "bed" for *hammock*).

C. Selection and Presentation of VCIU Stimuli

The stimuli for VCIU are chosen initially from the patient's own involuntary or spontaneously produced utterances. Ideally one should obtain a record of verbalizations produced in natural settings. More practically, the clinician should record every verbal utterance made by the patient during an interview and a comprehensive aphasia exam such as the *Boston Diagnostic Aphasia Examination* (BDAE). For example, one patient, Mr. N, produced the stereotypic expression "this and this" in conversation and for the "Cookie Theft" picture description. Occasionally he said "yes" and "no" in an unreliable manner. In the BDAE Word Repetition subtest he said "kiss" for *hammock* and "two" for *W.* In Confrontation Naming he said "die" for *chair.* He orally read *fifteen* as "three-five."

The clinician involved began Mr. N's first VCIU session by writing the words *kiss, die, two, three-five, yes,* and *no* on separate pieces of paper. These were presented to him one word at a time. Of the five words, he orally read *kiss, die,* and *two* correctly without struggle, so these were written separately in lowercase print on 3″ × 5″ index cards in bold, black ink. Because two of the spontaneously uttered words had emotional value, and because evidence (Landis, Graves, & Goodglass, 1982) indicates that severely aphasic patients orally read emotional words better than nonemotional ones, the patient was presented with two emotionally laden words: *love* and *war.* He read these correctly also, and they were printed separately on index cards. Next the clinician presented the word *father.* Mr. N read it as "mother," so *father* was discarded and the word *mother* was offered. He said "mama," so *mother* was discarded and "mama" was offered. He read this correctly, so *mama* was printed on an index card. The next stimulus, *milk,* elicited a neologistic response, so it was immediately discarded and the word *good* was offered instead, and so on. During the first session the clinician isolated eight words that Mr. N could read aloud correctly and without struggle. These words (printed in lowercase on separate index cards) then were given to him for independent practice.

At the next session the clinician reviewed these eight words with the patient, and when he struggled with *good,* it was removed from the list to be reintroduced at a later date. The clinician then turned the remaining seven cards over and drew pictures to represent the printed words (e.g., hearts for *love,* "2" for *two,* a figure of a coffin for *dead*). These pictures were used for confrontation naming, but when Mr. N displayed any problems, he was shown the printed word on the other side immediately. Then, choosing stimuli from the VCIU Master List (see this chapter's Appendix) and using the approach just discussed, the clinician began adding words to the patient's oral reading list.

In the third session Mr. N was asked to respond first to the pictured items presented the day before, then to read aloud his new words from session 2. For those that were read correctly without struggle or with immediate self-correction, pictures were drawn on the back for confrontation naming and so on.

By the fifth session the patient's wife reported that he was producing a few different words at home, and so these new words were presented in the VCIU format. When Mr. N's confrontation naming vocabulary reached 100 words, the clinician introduced at the beginning of the session conversation topics that would encourage the use of these words. For example, asking the patient what he did in the morning might elicit the words *breakfast, eggs, juice, coffee,* and so forth.

D. Criteria for Continuation of VCIU

It is almost immediately apparent if VCIU is worth pursuing with a particular aphasic patient. In the first session, the clinician will have been able to isolate at least a few words that the patient can read orally without notable struggle. At least one new word is added to each session. After a few sessions, the patient should be able to use some of these words for confrontation naming. Usually family members or caregivers will report hearing new utterances after about six or seven sessions, and these are added to the VCIU list. As in all other aphasia treatment approaches, some progress should be noted in each session. If this does not occur, then the clinician may not be using the approach properly, or VCIU may not be appropriate for that patient. Occasionally one sees patients who perseverate on a few of their VCIU words and so fail to progress with this method; these patients may be candidates, instead, for the Treatment of Aphasic Perseveration program, described in chapter 17.

For most patients, VCIU continues until the patient has accumulated between 200 and 300 words and short phrases he or she can use propositionally (oral reading, confrontation naming, and conversational usage). At that point, one begins to see a greater deblocking effect, with the patient expanding his or her own voluntarily controlled vocabulary for purposes of communication. Retesting should point the way to a more advanced method of rehabilitation.

E. Measuring the Effects of VCIU

Although formal aphasia tests may not capture the full extent of the language recovery with VCIU therapy, insurance companies and other involved parties demand that clinicians produce formal measures of response to a particular method. Because the VCIU candidate's greatest hinderance to communication is severe impairment of verbal expression, one must choose some standardized tests or subtests of speech output to measure VCIU effectiveness. Although the present authors have used the BDAE subtests of confrontation and responsive naming and the "Cookie Theft" picture description with our patients, subtests of other standardized exams (e.g., *Porch Index of Communicative Ability* Subtest I, "Tell me what you do with each of these") could serve the same purpose. Baseline measures on these tests are obtained before VCIU is introduced and then readministered after 15 sessions to chart generalization of effects. If the performance on the chosen formal measure(s) is not at least *qualitatively* better, at this point the clinician should reconsider the method. If improved test performance is seen, however, one can continue for another 15 sessions or until a 200–300 VCIU vocabulary has been achieved and then readminister the test(s). At this point the patient may have shown sufficient progress to warrant more extensive retesting to help determine new treatment directions.

References and Suggested Readings

Goda, S. (1962). Spontaneous speech, a primary source of therapy material. *Journal of Speech and Hearing Disorders, 27,* 190–192.

Helm, N.A., & Barresi, B. (1980). Voluntary Control of Involuntary Utterances: A treatment approach for severe aphasia. In R. Brookshire (ed.), *Clinical Aphasiology Conference Proceedings.* Minneapolis, MN: BRK.

Huber, M. (1944). A phonetic approach to the problem of perception in a case of Wernicke's aphasia. *Journal of Speech Disorders, 9,* 227–257.

Jackson, H. (1878). On the affections of speech from disease of the brain. *Brain, 1,* 304–330.

Landis, T., Graves, R., & Goodglass, H. (1982). Emotional value facilitates lexical output in aphasia. *Cortex, 18,* 105–112.

Sheehan, V. (1946). Rehabilitation of aphasics in an army hospital. *Journal of Speech Disorders, 11,* 149–157.

Vignolo, L.A. (1964). Evolution of aphasia and language rehabilitation: A retrospective exploratory study. *Cortex, 1,* 344–367.

Appendix: VCIU Master List

a

all right
apple
army

b

*ball
*baby
*bye
big
blue
Boston
box
by
breakfast
bridge
bug

c/k

*coke
*key
cake
call
car
care
cat
clothes
coat
cold
comb
come
cut
kick

ch

chair
cheese
chew
church

d

dammit
dance
dive
doctor

e

ears
eat
egg(s)

f

*four
fall
fine
fish

g

*go
*good
give

h

*ham
hello
hi
him
home

horse
hotdog

i

*I don't know
I
I think
ice

j

*juice

l

*love
*lunch

m

*milk
*Monday
*money
mad
man
map
maybe
me
more
much

n

*no
name
news
nice
nose

nothing

nurse

o

*okay

orange

out

p

paper

pen

r

round

run

s/sh

*see

*shoe

*show

school

seem

sit

sleep

snow

shame

sheep

shit

shower

shut

t/th

*tie

*time

*two

tea

ten

tire

TV

thanks

three

that's right

u

up

/w/

*one

*watch

*what

one time

war

warm

wash

what time

when

y

*yes

you

(Plus family names and personally relevant proper names)

*good starter words

15 Melodic Intonation Therapy

Over 200 years ago it was observed that a young man who had been rendered speechless following a blow to the head could nonetheless sing in the church choir. This startling phenomenon, the preserved ability to sing despite severe aphasia, can be seen by all who work with aphasic individuals. In 1942 the German neurologist Kurt Goldstein pointed out that there are aphasic patients who are able to pronounce words in song that they are unable to pronounce under other circumstances. This observation prompted clinicians to recommend the use of music and rhythm in treatment of aphasia.

The American neurologist Charles Mills (1904), for example, suggested that it might be beneficial to play the piano and encourage patients to sing popular songs. It seems, however, that while this activity may benefit the patient psychologically, it may have little effect on propositional or conversational speech skills. Experience indicates that it is difficult to dissociate words strongly associated with a particular tune. In fact, everyone has experienced the difficulty of recalling words to a song if that song is begun at some midpoint instead of at the beginning where the words tumble forth in a highly automatic manner. Similarly, an aphasic patient is unlikely to have the capacity for extracting a word from a familiar song and using that word for purposeful communication.

It was the speech pathologist Ollie Backus (1945) who suggested presenting useful words and phrases to aphasic patients in a rhythmical, unison fashion. Not until 1972, however, was a formal study of such an approach undertaken. At that time Albert, Sparks, and Helm began to explore the use of a singing technique to facilitate and stimulate the propositional speech of severely nonfluent patients. In addition to clinical experience with patients who produced words only when singing, we were encouraged by emerging research evidence that the right cerebral hemisphere was important in mediating music. Hypothesizing that functions associated with the intact right hemisphere may be exploited for purposes of rehabilitating speech in left-brain-damaged individuals, we developed the technique now known as Melodic Intona-

tion Therapy, or MIT. (The name was first suggested by Sheila Blumstein, whose own research first identified the role of the right hemisphere in processing the intonational contours of spoken sentences.) In
1973 the first description was published of the effects of Melodic Intonation Therapy on three severely but not globally aphasic patients (see
Albert, Sparks, & Helm, 1973), followed the next year by a study of eight
patients who had shown no improvement in verbal expression (despite
other therapy) before entering the MIT program (see Sparks, Helm, &
Albert, 1974). Six of the eight had notable improvement in propositional
speech with MIT.

A. The Melodic Intonation Therapy Program

Melodic Intonation Therapy is a hierarchically structured program that is divided into three levels. In the first two levels,
multisyllabic words and short, high-probability phrases are
musically intoned. The third level introduces longer or more
phonologically complex sentences. These longer sentences first
are intoned, then produced with exaggerated speech prosody,
and finally spoken normally. On all intoned phrases the clinician taps the patient's left hand once for each syllable. Items
are intoned *very slowly, with continuous voicing,* using simple
high note–low note patterns based on the normal speech prosody of the phrase.

B. Candidacy for MIT

Two studies (Helm, 1978; Naeser & Helm-Estabrooks, 1985)
have been directed specifically at identifying those patients
who will respond best to MIT as measured by the *Boston Diagnostic Aphasia Examination.* Good response is defined as
improvement in conversational speech skills following a course
of MIT and not as the ability simply to complete the program.
Patients with good repetition, for example, may be able to progress through the MIT hierarchy but show little or no improvement in their ability to verbally communicate. Patients who
will show good response to MIT have most of all of the following
characteristics:

Pre-treatment characteristics of good MIT candidates:

1. **Etiology:** unilateral, left-hemisphere stroke.

2. **Lesion:** confined to the left cerebral hemisphere and
   involving Broca's area, or undercutting Broca's area with

inclusion of periventricular white matter deep to lower motor cortex for face.

3. **Speech output:** poorly articulated, nonfluent, or severely restricted verbal output that may be confined to a nonsense stereotypy (e.g., "bika bika").

4. **Auditory comprehension:** at least moderately preserved, exceeding the 45th percentile on the BDAE Rating Scale.

5. **Repetition:** poor, even for single words.

6. **Articulation:** poorly articulated speech, earning a rating of 3 or less on the BDAE Profile of Speech Characteristics.

7. **Psychological features:** well motivated, emotionally stable, with good attention span.

These candidacy studies also have identified the characteristics of patients with poor response to Melodic Intonation Therapy. Some of these patients actually were able to complete the MIT program but showed no changes in their communicative speech skills as a result of this form of treatment. The characteristics of these poor-response cases follow:

Pre-treatment characteristics of poor MIT candidates:

1. **Etiology:** closed head trauma, bilateral strokes/surgery.

2. **Lesion:** bilateral lesions, or large lesion in Wernicke's area or left temporal isthmus.

3. **Speech output:** moderately to well-articulated speech, with a phrase length of four or more words.

4. **Auditory comprehension:** relatively poor, earning an overall score of less than 45% on the BDAE Rating Scale.

5. **Repetition:** good repetition for at least multisyllabic words.

6. **Articulation:** normal for at least familiar words and phrases, earning a score of 4 or more on the BDAE Profile of Speech Characteristics.

7. **Psychological features:** emotionally unstable and/or pseudobulbar affect, poorly motivated, poor attention span.

C. **Preparing for an MIT Session**

Melodic Intonation Therapy requires preselected stimulus items with corresponding pictures and an MIT score sheet (see

Helm-Estabrooks, Nicholas, & Morgan, 1989). MIT is administered with the clinician and patient seated across from one another at a table. The use of the tabletop is important for hand tapping.

Stimulus items should be high probability words (of at least two syllables), phrases, and sentences. In selecting these items, phonological difficulty and number of syllables should be considered. For example, it is best to avoid consonant blends and to favor visualizable (e.g., bilabials) sounds in the first level. Similarly, the clinician should attend to syntactic complexity. Imperative sentences (e.g. "Sit down"; "Open the door") often are easiest in the earlier stages. (The hierarchy of syntactic difficulty used in the HELPSS program described in chapter 16 may provide a guideline for selection items.) Naturally, the communication needs of the individual patient also must be considered when choosing items. The use of family names, for example, may be helpful.

If at all possible, each intoned item should be accompanied by pictures or environmental cues to increase saliency. Further, it is important to have a wide selection of words, phrases, and sentences to be rotated through a series of treatment sessions. The use of a limited set of stimuli fails to provide a therapeutic level of language stimulation and may induce perseveration. Perseveration can be further avoided by alternating items according to the pitch patterns or number of syllables. For example, two successive items with a two-syllable, high/low pitch pattern may induce perseveration and should be separated by a three-syllable word that has a different pitch pattern.

D. Presentation of Items

Each word, phrase, or sentence should be intoned *slowly*, with constant voicing, using high/low tones and the stress and rhythm patterns associated with normal speech. It is best to determine the pitch, stress, and rhythm patterns before beginning the session (see Fig. 15.1 for some examples). Sit directly across from the patient so that he or she can see your face/mouth, and note how the sounds are formed. Hold the patient's left hand with your right hand and tap once for each intoned syllable; use your left hand to signal the patient when to listen and when to intone. At all times a staccato approach should be avoided, as it is the continuous voicing that facilitates verbal production.

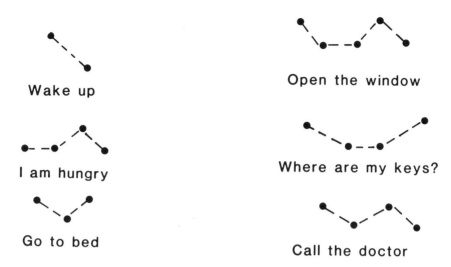

FIG. 15.1. Melodic Intonation Therapy: sample pitch patterns

E. Overview of the Scoring Procedure

For items presented in Level I, a score of 0 or 1 can be earned at each step. For items at Levels II or III, scores of 0, 1, or 2 are possible. In general, a full score is earned at each step if the patient is successful. (The clinician may set different criteria for what is considered "successful" according to individual patients. For example, if a patient with severe dysarthria, who is otherwise unintelligible, produces an intelligible version of the target response when intoning, then that may be considered "successful".) For items that allow for "backups," a patient may earn partial credit (a score of 1) if he or she succeeds with the aid of the backup. As a rule of thumb, any item not adequately produced after four repetitions at a particular step is discontinued and a score of 0 is recorded. The specific target scores for each step and level are outlined as follows:

1. **Scoring each session and advancing to higher levels.** In order to record the patient's progress in Melodic Intonation Therapy, session score sheets are necessary. Graph paper can be used to track session-by-session progress and to determine discontinuation, advancement to a higher level, or ultimate discharge. To calculate the overall score for each session using 10 or more stimulus items, the following procedure is adopted:

a. Add the total points earned for each step (one column for each step).

b. Count the number of possible points that could be earned for each step (i.e., the number of items presented × the number of points that could be earned for that step).

c. Divide the sum of #1 (total points earned) by #2 (total possible points that could be earned) and multiply by 100 to yield the percent correct performance at each step.

d. Sum the numbers of earned points for all steps and divide by the sum of possible points for all steps. Multiply by 100 to calculate the overall percentage sum for the entire session.

2. **Criteria for continuation and advancement.** To remain in the Melodic Intonation Therapy program, the average score for three sessions must be higher than the average score for the three preceding sessions, using a variety of stimulus items. To progress from one level of MIT to the next, the patient must earn an overall score of 90% or better for five consecutive sessions using a variety of stimuli.

F. Level-by-Level and Step-by-Step Procedures

MIT Level I consists of five steps, the first of which is not scored. There is no interruption *between* the steps for scoring; one stimulus item is carried through as many of the five steps as possible before a new item is introduced. Each of the four scorable steps (2–5) is worth 1 point. If the primary goal of a particular step is not achieved for any item, that item is discontinued and the next item is introduced at step 1. Assisted hand tapping accompanies each production of the target phrase; that is, the clinician picks up the patient's left hand and taps it on the tabletop once for each syllable of the target phrase. Pictures or environmental cues related to the target items are referred to throughout to enhance the saliency of the words or phrases. Descriptions of the five steps that make up Level I follow:

1. **Humming.** Begin by humming the melody pattern of the target item while referring to a picture or environmental cue related to the target. Then intone (sing) the item twice,

using a high note/low note approach according to the natural pitch and stress pattern of a particular item. The patient is required merely to attend and allow his or her hand to be tapped. Because no response is required, no score is possible.

2. **Unison singing.** Intone the target phrase in unison with the patient, again with assisted hand tapping. If the patient has not produced the item with acceptable intelligibility after four repetitions, drop the item and record a score of 0. Then introduce a new item at step 1. If the patient's performance is acceptable, introduce step 3.

3. **Unison with fading.** Intone and tap the target phrase in unison with the patient, but about halfway through the item fade out so the patient must complete the item alone. Do not lip-sync the item once you have faded out; this provides a strong cue to patients who otherwise may be unable to complete the item.

4. **Immediate repetition.** Intone and tap the target phrase while the patient listens. Immediately following this, let the patient intone the phrase in repetition and assist with hand tapping. (It is helpful to use your left hand to signal the patient when to just listen and when to intone.) If the patient is successful, record a score of 1 and introduce step 5.

5. **Response to a probe question.** Immediately following successful repetition, quickly intone an appropriate probe question (e.g., "What did you say?"). No hand tapping accompanies the quickly intoned probe question; the only assistance the patient may receive in answering the question is hand-tapping the syllable pattern of the target phrase. If the patient succeeds in producing the target phrase in response to the question, assign a score of 1 and introduce a new target phrase at step 1.

MIT Level II introduces "delays" between stimulus and response. In order to help the patient respond correctly after a delay, "backups" are used; that is, if a patient is unable to complete a step with delays, he or she is permitted to back up to a previous step. Steps with potential backups (3 and 4) are worth 2 points; however, if the patient must use a backup to succeed, only 1 point is awarded. If a patient does not succeed even with a backup, the clinician records a score of 0 and a new item is introduced. As in Level I, each target phrase is intoned and accompanied by hand tapping.

Unison with fading should be repeated twice even if the patient is initially successful. Up to four attempts to achieve the target behavior are allowed; if the patient succeeds, 1 point is earned and the next step is introduced. Once again, if the patient fails, the item is dropped and a new item is introduced at step 1. Descriptions of the four steps at Level II follow:

1. **Introduction of item.** Intone the target phrase twice while tapping the patient's hand. As in Level I, the use of related pictures or environmental cues is encouraged. No response is required, *so no score is possible.*

2. **Unison with fading.** Begin intoning and tapping the target phrase in unison with the patient, but at about the halfway point fade out, leaving the patient to complete the item. If the patient fails, discontinue the item and introduce a new item at step 1. If the patient succeeds, record 1 point and introduce step 3.

3. **Delayed repetition.** Intone and tap the target phrase. After approximately 6 seconds of delay, help the patient tap the item, but then allow him or her to intone the words *without verbal assistance.* If he or she succeeds, then score 2 points and introduce step 4. If the patient fails, back up to step 2. If the backup is successful, attempt delayed repetition once again. Should the patient fail this time, discontinue the phrase and introduce a new item at step 1. If he or she succeeds, then record 1 point and begin step 4 *following a 6-second delay.*

4. **Response to a probe question.** After waiting approximately 6 seconds following successful completion of step 3, quickly intone a probe question (e.g., "What did you say?"). No hand tapping accompanies this question, which merely elicits the target response from the patient who intones the item alone. If he or she succeeds, 2 points are earned. If the patient fails, back up to step 3. Six seconds after a successful completion of the backup, again intone the probe question. If the patient fails to respond with the target this time, discontinue the item for a score of 0 and introduce a new item at step 1. If the patient succeeds with the backup, record 1 point.

MIT Level III is designed to return the speech of the patient to normal prosody, using more complex target sentences. This is achieved through a transitional technique called **sprech-gesang** or "speech song." In this technique the rhythm and stress of each target phrase are accentuated while the intonational characteristics used in previous levels are dropped and replaced by the constantly changing pitch of normal speech, much like choral speaking. Four of the five steps in Level III can be scored. Each is worth 2 points if backups are not required; 1 point is awarded if success follows use of a backup. Failure to achieve a step's primary task earns a score of 0. Descriptions of the five Level III steps follow:

1. **Delayed repetition.** Tap and intone the target phrase. After a 6-second delay, let the patient intone the phrase once in repetition. The only assistance allowable is hand tapping. If the patient succeeds, record 2 points; if he or she fails, introduce a backup. Intone the phrase in unison with the patient, then fade, leaving the patient to complete the item alone. Following successful completion of the backup, attempt delayed repetition again. Success at this point earns 1 point, and step 2 is introduced. If the patient fails after a backup, record a score of 0 and introduce a new item.

2. **Introducing sprechgesang.** Present the target phrase twice in sprechgesang. Do not sing the words, but rather present them slowly with exaggerated rhythm and stress, as in choral speaking. Accompany this by hand tapping. No response is required, so *no score is possible.*

3. **Sprechgesang with fading.** Begin the item together with the patient in sprechgesang, but then fade, leaving the patient to complete the phrase alone. If the patient succeeds, record 2 points; if he or she fails, then try full unison presentation without fading. If this is successful, attempt step 3 again. Successful performance following backup earns 1 point, and step 4 is introduced. Score an unsuccessful performance after a backup as 0 and introduce a new item at step 1.

4. **Delayed spoken repetition.** Present the item in normal speech prosody *without hand tapping.* After a 6-second delay, let the patient repeat the item using normal speech prosody. If he or she succeeds, score 2 points. If the patient fails, back up to step 3, then attempt step 4 again. Successful performance following the backup earns 1 point.

TABLE 15.1
Overview of Melodic Intonation Therapy

Level	Step	No. of points
I.	1. Humming	no score
	2. Unison singing	1
	3. Unison singing with fading	1
	4. Immediate repetition	1
	5. Response to a probe question	1
II.	1. Introduction of item	no score
	2. Unison with fading	1
	3. Delayed repetition	2
	(*Backup:* Unison with fading)	1
	4. Response to probe question	2
	(*Backup:* Delayed repetition)	1
III.	1. Delayed repetition	2
	(*Backup:* Unison with fading)	1
	2. Introducing sprechgesang	no score
	3. Sprechgesang with fading	2
	(*Backup:* Unison sprechgesang)	1
	4. Spoken repetition with delay	2
	(*Backup:* Sprechgesang with fading)	1
	5. Response to probe question	2
	(*Backup:* Delayed repetition)	1

Begin step 5 after a 6-second delay. Score an unsuccessful performance after a backup as 0 and introduce a new item.

5. **Response to a probe question.** After a 6-second delay, ask an appropriate probe question with normal speech prosody. The patient must respond with the normally spoken target phrase. If he or she succeeds, record 2 points; if he or she fails, back up to step 4, and then attempt step 5 again. If the patient now is successful, score 1 point and introduce a new item at step 1. Score an unsuccessful performance after a backup as 0 and introduce a new item.

A summary of the Melodic Intonation Therapy procedure appears in Table 15.1.

G. Measuring Response to MIT

The ultimate goal of Melodic Intonation Therapy is to improve the verbal communication skills of patients with restricted speech output. The MIT program can only be judged successful if it has a significantly positive effect on conversational speech skills. Some patients, such as those with transcortical motor aphasia, may have the ability to complete MIT (the independent variable) without showing changes on some dependent measure of the target behavior (the dependent variable). It is helpful to tape-record both conversational and expository speech samples to measure response to MIT. Using these tape-recorded samples, one can judge the patient on both conversational speech/language parameters and the "Cookie Theft" picture performance measure described in chapter 11. The following offers an example of how this method can be used to measure a patient's response to MIT:

Pre-MIT

9/29: "A (unintelligible) getting (unintelligible) . . . . An the ink wrinning ower . . . um . . . giffle *boy* came (unintelligible) . . . boother . . . uh . . . sister (unintelligible)."

12 words   1 bound morpheme   4 content units

Index of Lexical Efficiency = 3.0

Index of Grammatical Support = 2.3

Post-MIT

12/11: "The wady is doing her dishes. Link under over . . . uh. The window is open and co-son . . . a very funny day outside. Children . . . a boy and a girl. The boy is up on a stoop and is stealing cookies and pass'em to . . . to his sister. I uh . . . I see nothing un-us-u-al about the picture."

15 words   13 content units   4 bound morphemes

Index of Lexical Efficiency = 4.0

Index of Grammatical Support = 2.4

References and Suggested Readings

Albert, M., Sparks, R., & Helm, N. (1973). Melodic Intonation Therapy for aphasia. *Archives of Neurology, 29,* 130–131.

Backus, O. (1945). The rehabilitation of persons with aphasia. In *The rehabilitation of speech.* New York: Harper Bros.

Goldstein, K. (1942). *After effects of brain-injuries in war: Their evaluation and treatment.* New York: Grune & Stratton.

Helm, N.A. (1978, February). *Criteria for selecting aphasic patients for Melodic Intonation Therapy.* Paper presented at the meeting of the American Academy for the Advancement of Science, Washington, DC.

Helm-Estabrooks, N., Nicholas, M., & Morgan, A. (1989). *Melodic Intonation Therapy program.* San Antonio, TX: Special Press.

Mills, C.K. (1904). Treatment of aphasia by training. *Journal of the American Medical Association, 43,* 1940–1949.

Naeser, M., & Helm-Estabrooks, N. (1985). CT scan lesion localization and response to Melodic Intonation Therapy with nonfluent aphasia cases. *Cortex, 21,* 203–223.

Sparks, R., Helm, N., & Albert, M. (1974). Aphasia rehabilitation resulting from Melodic Intonation Therapy. *Cortex, 10,* 303–316.

16

Helm Elicited Program for Syntax Stimulation

Two forms of grammatical disorder have been described in association with aphasia: **paragrammatism** and **agrammatism**. Paragrammatism occurs in fluent aphasia and is characterized by grammatical errors such as incorrect tense markers or misuse of pronouns in the context of a wide range of syntactic constructions. Agrammatism occurs in non-fluent aphasia and is characterized by the production of mostly substantive words or short phrases in which functor words such as articles, prepositions, personal pronouns, and verb inflections are omitted. Of the two forms of grammatical disorder, agrammatism typically poses a far greater problem for communication; further, agrammatic patients may comprise a large portion of the language clinician's aphasia caseload. For these reasons, treatment of agrammatism has received more attention than the treatment of paragrammatism.

In general, programs for agrammatism have been based on such factors as ease of syntax comprehension for normals, language acquisition models, or approaches to teaching English as a second language. However, we believe that treatment should be based on a careful analysis of the patient's own strengths and weaknesses, so for treatment of agrammatism we turned to a study of agrammatism carried out by Gleason, Goodglass, Green, Ackerman, and Hyde (1975). In this study, a story completion technique was used to elicit spoken examples of 14 syntactic constructions from eight patients with Broca's aphasia and agrammatism. For example, to elicit an imperative intransitive sentence the examiner might say, "My friend comes in. I want him to sit down, so I say to him what?", and the patient responds with "Sit down." An order of difficulty was found across the 14 constructions, with imperative intransitive statements the easiest and future tense sentences the most difficult for agrammatic patients to produce. But despite this hierarchy of difficulty, even the most severely agrammatic patient produced at least one correct or nearly correct response for each construction. The investigators concluded that patients have an impaired and inconsistent access to syntactic knowledge rather than a lack of that knowledge.

These results suggested that, with practice, agrammatic patients may improve in their ability to produce a wide variety of syntax for purposes of communication. It is axiomatic in aphasia treatment to begin where the patient is most likely to succeed with little struggle and to progress in small increments of difficulty. In keeping with this philosophy, Helm (unpublished study) based a program on the hierarchy of difficulty found in the 1975 study, beginning with the imperative intransitive. Not only was order of difficulty incorporated, but the story completion technique was adopted and modified to provide the patient with two levels of difficulty. Two additional modifications involved adding pictures to reinforce each stimulus item, and omitting the three nonsentence phrase forms used in the 1975 study. This program, first called the Syntax Stimulation Program (Helm-Estabrooks, Fitzpatrick, & Barresi, 1981), subsequently was named Helm Elicited Program for Syntax Stimulation, or HELPSS (Helm-Estabrooks, 1981).

More recently, the results of a group study of six long-term agrammatic patients has demonstrated the efficacy of HELPSS (Helm-Estabrooks & Ramsberger, 1986b). In these cases, patients treated with HELPSS showed significant positive changes in conversational phrase length, *Boston Diagnostic Aphasia Examination* (BDAE) "Cookie Theft" picture description, and *Northwestern Syntax Screening Test* (Lee, 1969) expressive scores. Furthermore, HELPSS has been used effectively via telephone to treat patients who are unable to come to the clinic (Helm-Estabrooks & Ramsberger, 1986a).

A. The Helm Elicited Program for Syntax Stimulation

The Helm Elicited Program for Syntax Stimulation is a hierarchically structured approach to therapy that uses a story completion format to elicit 11 sentence types. There are two task levels (A and B) and multiple exemplars for each syntactic construction. Each exemplar is accompanied by a simple line drawing (see Fig. 16.1).

In Level A, the clinician reads a short story (usually about two sentences in length) that ends with the target sentence. The story then is reread without the target sentence, which must be supplied by the patient. When Level A has been completed for a particular sentence type, using a 90% accuracy criterion for success, the second level is introduced. In Level B the story does not contain the target sentence. Instead, the patient must produce the target as a logical completion of the story, but without the benefit of having heard the target as part of the stimulus. When score criterion has been reached for Sentence Type 1,

LEVEL A

Probe: Rob's grandchild is bored. Rob gets a book, and he reads
                      his grandchild a story. What does he do?

Target Response: He reads his grandchild a story.

LEVEL B

Probe: Rob's grandchild is bored. Rob gets a book, and what does
                      he do?

Target Response: He reads his grandchild a story.

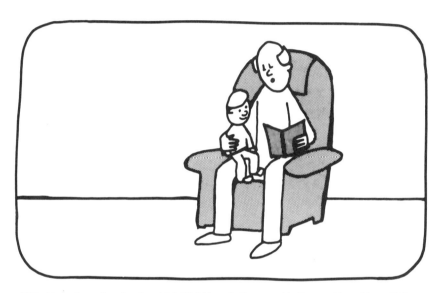

FIG. 16.1. Sample stimulus: HELPSS Type 9 direct and indirect object (From *Helm Elicited Program for Syntax Stimulation* by Nancy Helm-Estabrooks. Copyright 1981 by PRO-ED, Inc. Reprinted by permission.)

Level B, the patient is introduced to Sentence Type 2 at Level A, and so on until he or she can produce all 11 types at both levels of difficulty.

Although HELPSS is a highly structured approach, it is important to acknowledge that no single approach can or should be applied strictly to each patient. For example, some patients may find Sentence Type 9 (Direct and Indirect Object; e.g., "He gives his son a toy") more difficult than Sentence Type 11

(Future; e.g., "He will sleep"). Other patients may have to complete all sentence types at Level A before progressing to Level B. Similarly, certain words may prove difficult for individual patients. In administering a program like HELPSS, the clinician must not lose sight of the purpose of the program, which is to stimulate and facilitate grammatical speech and not to teach rigid and rote verbal output. To that end, the clinician has a responsibility to modify the program according to the performance needs of a particular patient.

B. Candidacy for HELPSS

HELPSS is a program for aphasic patients who display agrammatism and moderate to well-preserved auditory comprehension. It is *not* appropriate for patients with little or no speech output or severely impaired auditory comprehension. For a diagnosis of agrammatism, the patient must produce conversational and expository speech that consists mainly of substantive words, with little use of functors and grammatical inflections. For example, the following "Cookie Theft" picture descriptions was elicited from a patient who proved to be a good candidate for HELPSS: "Water. Girl . . . down. Washing dishes. She got . . . cookie. Fall down. He got cookie." Time post onset has not been an important factor in determining positive response to HELPSS, if the patient otherwise has the following characteristics:

Pre-treatment characteristics of good HELPSS candidates:

1. **Etiology:** unilateral, left-hemisphere stroke.

2. **Lesion:** confined to the left cerebral hemisphere, usually sparing posterior language zones.

3. **Aphasia type:** Broca's aphasia, transcortical motor aphasia, anterior capsular/putaminal aphasia.

4. **Speech output:** nonfluent with restricted grammatical form and average phrase length of two to five words, consisting mainly of substantive words.

5. **Auditory comprehension:** good single-word comprehension and fair to good comprehension for sentences and paragraphs.

6. **Psychological features:** may be frustrated by restricted ability to communicate but is cooperative, displays good

attention span and memory, and appreciates the goal of the program.

C. Preparing for a HELPSS Session

Although the HELPSS program is available as a published package (Helm-Estabrooks, 1981), a clinician may want to custom design a program for a particular patient using stimuli relevant to the patient's life-style and communication needs. In any case, it is important to have a variety of exemplars for each construction to stimulate the patient maximally. Prior to each session, the clinician should prepare a set of stimulus stories for at least two sentence types so that flexibility can be maintained if the patient shows notable difficulty or ease with a certain construction or exemplar. One should accompany each story/exemplar with a related picture to increase the saliency of the spoken stimuli.

Before the patient is introduced to the program, baseline measures of syntactic skills should be obtained. This can be accomplished via a conversational speech sample, the BDAE "Cookie Theft" picture description, and the *Northwestern Syntax Screening Test,* which has measures of both receptive and expressive skills.

D. The Scoring Procedure

Although it is important to record the patient's exact response to each story completion probe, a simple 3-point scoring system determines progress from one level to another and from one sentence type to another: 1.0 = a fully correct response, .5 = a self-corrected response, and 0 = an incomplete or incorrect response. The criterion for progression from one step to another is a score of 90% of the highest possible score. For example, if one uses 20 exemplars of Sentence Type 5, Declarative Intransitive, then the patient must earn an overall score of 18 or better at Level A in order to progress to Level B, and an overall score of 18 or better at Level B in order to progress to the Comparative construction (Sentence Type 6).

If multiple trials are required for any sentence construction, then the average score for any three trials should be higher than the average score for three previous trials or the clinician should question the appropriateness of the HELPSS program for that patient. At the same time, all error responses should be recorded and analyzed between each session to determine both the nature of the problem and whether any program modifications are required.

E. HELPSS Sentence Types and Levels

As stated previously, HELPSS consists of 11 sentence types, each presented at two levels of difficulty with multiple exemplars of each type elicited by story completion probes. Pictures, but not written sentences, accompany each story. Approximately 20 stories and exemplars of each construction are presented, usually in the following order of difficulty (sample exchanges between clinician and patient appear for each):

1. Sentence Type 1—Imperative Intransitive

Level A: (Clinician) "My friend feels dizzy, so I tell him, 'Lie down.' What do I tell him?"

(Patient) "Lie down."

Level B: (Clinician) "My friend feels dizzy, so I tell him what?"

(Patient) "Lie down."

2. Sentence Type 2—Imperative Transitive

Level A: (Clinician) "When supper is over, I say to my roommate, 'Wash the dishes.' What do I say?"

(Patient) "Wash the dishes."

Level B: (Clinician) "Supper is over, so I say to my roommate what?"

(Patient) "Wash the dishes."

3. Sentence Type 3—*Wh-* Interrogative

Level A: (Clinician) "When I see my friend sitting at her word processor, I say, 'What are you writing?' What do I say?"

(Patient) "What are you writing?"

Level B: (Clinician) "Whenever I see my friend sitting at her word processor, I say to her what?"

(Patient) "What are you writing?"

4. Sentence Type 4—Declarative Transitive

Level A: (Clinician) "When people ask me what my friend does for a living, I tell them, 'She cleans teeth.' What do I tell them?"

(Patient) "She cleans teeth."

Level B: (Clinician) "When people ask me what my friend does for a living, I tell them what?"

(Patient) "She cleans teeth."

5. Sentence Type 5—Declarative Intransitive

Level A: (Clinician) "When my cousin goes to the ice rink, she skates. What does she do?"

(Patient) "She skates."

Level B: (Clinician) "When my cousin goes to the rink, she does what?"

(Patient) "She skates."

6. Sentence Type 6—Comparative

Level A: (Clinician) "No one ever laughs at Hal's jokes, but everyone laughs at Mick's because they're funnier. Everyone laughs at Mick's jokes. How come?"

(Patient) "They're funnier."

Level B: (Clinician) "No one ever laughs at Hal's jokes, but everyone laughs at Mick's jokes because . . . ?"

(Patient) "They're funnier."

7. Sentence Type 7—Passive

Level A: (Clinician) "The baggage tag fell off my luggage and the suitcases were lost. What happened?"

(Patient) "The suitcases were lost."

Level B: (Clinician) "The baggage tag fell off my luggage and what happened?"

(Patient) "The suitcases were lost."

8. **Sentence Type 8—Yes/No Questions**

Level A: (Clinician) "Linda wonders whether her husband bought the paper, so she asks, 'Did you buy the paper?' What did she ask?"

(Patient) "Did you buy the paper?"

Level B: (Clinician) "Linda wonders whether her husband bought the paper, so she says what?"

(Patient) "Did you buy the paper?"

9. **Sentence Type 9—Direct and Indirect Object**

Level A: (Clinician) "It's Pat's birthday. Her friends want to celebrate, so they give Pat a cake. What do they do?"

(Patient) "They give Pat a cake."

Level B: (Clinician) "It's Pat's birthday and her friends want to celebrate, so what do they do?"

(Patient) "They give Pat a cake."

10. **Sentence Type 10—Embedded Sentences**

Level A: (Clinician) "Dave was always eating junk food. His mother was concerned. She wanted him to be healthy. Why was she concerned?"

(Patient) "She wanted him to be healthy."

Level B: (Clinician) "Dave was eating too much junk food. His mother was concerned because . . . ?"

(Patient) "She wanted him to be healthy."

11. **Sentence Type 11—Future**

Level A: (Clinician) "Whenever my friend goes to the mountains, he hikes. Next month he is visiting the Alps, so he will hike. What will happen?"

(Patient) "He will hike."

Level B: (Clinician) "Whenever my friend goes to the mountains, he hikes. Next month he is visiting the Alps, so what will happen?"

(Patient) "He will hike."

F. Measuring Response to HELPSS

The best measure of the effectiveness of a program for improving language output in aphasia is the extent to which the patient improves in functional, everyday verbal communication. It is often difficult for the clinician to capture this, however, as the communication between patient and clinician tends to be circumscribed. Instead one must rely on formal test measures and informal reports from those who interact with the patient in more natural settings. One method useful for documenting the patient's functional communication is to give a family member or primary caregiver a notebook and ask them to record new utterances heard during the treatment period.

The clinician always should obtain a conversational and expository speech sample before and after treatment and usually at a halfway point. It is beneficial to analyze the BDAE "Cookie Theft" picture description according to the method described in chapter 11 and look for positive changes in content units, the Index of Grammatical Support, and the Index of Lexical Efficiencies.

In addition, the *Northwestern Syntax Screening Test* (NSST) is recommended. The NSST uses pictures and sentence stimuli to obtain both a receptive measure of syntax comprehension and an expressive measure of syntactical verbal production. An all or none scoring system awards 1 point for each correct response. But because this system may fail to capture the extent to which verbal production may improve with HELPSS, one should analyze each verbal response according to the number of correct target morphemes produced. For example, for the sentence "The girl sees the dog," one patient may simply say "Dog" before HELPSS treatment and "The girl are seeing the dog" after treatment. Although both responses earn an NSST score of 0, the correct morpheme score was 1 before treatment and 5 afterward.

Research with HELPSS indicates that a good candidate for this method will show significant improvement in both content units and grammatical morphemes on the "Cookie Theft" picture description and significant improvement in expressive raw scores and correct target morphemes on the NSST. Furthermore, these improvements on formal tests appear to reflect the patient's ability to produce a greater variety of grammatical forms in conversation.

References and Suggested Readings

Gleason, J.B., Goodglass, H., Green, E., Ackerman, N., & Hyde, M. (1975). The retrieval of syntax in Broca's aphasia. *Brain and Language, 24,* 451–457.

Helm-Estabrooks, N., Fitzpatrick, P., & Barresi, B. (1981). Response of an agrammatic patient to a syntax program for aphasia. *Journal of Speech and Hearing Disorders, 46,* 422–427.

Helm-Estabrooks, N. (1981). *Helm Elicited Language Program for Syntax Stimulation.* Austin, TX: PRO-ED.

Helm-Estabrooks, N., & Ramsberger, G. (1986a). Aphasia treatment delivered by telephone. *Archives of Physical Medicine and Rehabilitation, 67,* 51–53.

Helm-Estabrooks, N., & Ramsberger, G. (1986b). Treatment of agrammatism in long-term Broca's aphasia. *British Journal of Disorders of Communication, 21,* 39–45.

Lee, L. (1969). *Northwestern Syntax Screening Test.* Evanston, IL: Northwestern University Press.

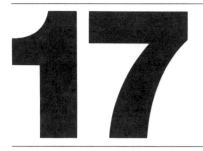

Treatment of Aphasic Perseveration

Perseveration is one of the most common behavioral disorders associated with aphasia. The term refers to the inappropriate continuation or recurrence of an earlier response after the task requirement has changed. As briefly described in chapter 7, perseveration manifests itself in at least three forms in aphasia: (a) the **stuck-in-set** variety, defined as the inappropriate maintenance of a category or framework of response (e.g., on the *Boston Diagnostic Aphasia Examination* [BDAE] Following Commands subtest, pointing to the head and feet instead of the ceiling and floor because the previous subtest required pointing to parts of the body); (b) the **continuous** variety, defined as the inappropriate prolongation or continuation of a behavior without cessation (e.g., a patient who continues to place loops on the number 3 as he attempts to write his address); and (c) the **recurrent** variety, defined as the inappropriate occurrence of a previous response following the intervening presentation of a new stimulus (e.g., in naming consecutive colors, a patient says "brown" for *brown,* "pink" for *pink,* and then "brown" for *blue*).

Of the three varieties of perseveration, recurrent perseveration is the type most frequently seen in aphasia. Furthermore, tests of confrontation naming are most likely to elicit recurrent perseveration, with variables such as word frequency, word length, phonemic complexity, and semantic class influencing the severity of perseverative behavior.

To examine the role of perseveration in confrontation naming, Emery and Helm-Estabrooks (1989) looked at the naming responses of 30 aphasic patients (15 fluent and 15 nonfluent) on the BDAE Confrontation Naming subtest, which is comprised of items from seven semantic categories. The patients represented a variety of aphasia syndromes and ranged in severity of naming deficits. The study found that all 30 subjects demonstrated perseverative behavior on this subtest, and the incidence of perseveration was significantly but negatively correlated with the naming score. For 26 patients, at least 35% of their naming errors were perseverations. Severity of perseveration was not related either to time post onset or the fluent/nonfluent aphasia classification.

These results supported Albert and Sandson's (1986) contention that perseveration is an integral part of aphasia, suggesting that one approach to aphasia rehabilitation might be to deblock language performance by directly addressing perseverative behaviors. In an attempt to accomplish this, the Treatment of Aphasic Perseveration, or TAP, program was developed (Helm-Estabrooks, Emery, & Albert, 1987). The program was administered to three patients displaying moderate to severe perseveration on the BDAE naming subtest. Each patient was treated using an ABAB design in which TAP was alternated with another treatment in five session blocks. For all three, the TAP program was significantly more effective than the alternative therapies in reducing perseveration. Further, as perseveration diminished, naming scores improved substantially. Since the publication of this study, we have replicated these results with several other patients demonstrating moderate to severe perseveration on the BDAE Confrontation Naming subtest.

A. The Treatment of Aphasic Perseveration Program

The TAP program was developed for patients who manifest at least a moderate degree of perseveration on tests of confrontation naming. TAP uses the same seven semantic categories as the *Boston Diagnostic Aphasia Examination* (Objects, Letters, Geometric Forms, Actions, Numbers, Colors, and Body Parts). The TAP items, however, are different from those on the BDAE and were chosen on the basis of frequency of use, concreteness, word length, phonetic and semantic variability, and emotionality (see the Appendix to this chapter for an item listing). Where possible, real objects are used in addition to pictures of each item. Each item is shown to the patient for confrontation naming according to a predetermined order, based on the strengths and weaknesses displayed by that patient on the BDAE. If the patient cannot name an item, as many as three of the cues may be used to elicit a correct response. After naming the item correctly with a cue, however, the patient must immediately name to confrontation (i.e., "So what is this?"). The ultimate goal of the program is for the patient to name 90% (34/38) of the pictured stimuli with perseverations occurring on no more than 10% (or 4) of the items (progress is charted on graphs noting correct responses, number of cues, and perseverations). If the patient does not show a pattern of diminishing perseveration with improved naming over five session blocks of treatment, then TAP is discontinued.

B. Candidacy for the TAP Program

Patients who show a moderate to severe degree of perseveration in confrontation naming may be good candidates for TAP. In order to determine severity of perseveration, a two-step procedure can be followed:

1. Administer the BDAE Confrontation Naming subtest. Use checkmarks only for responses that are correct without false attempts. Transcribe all incorrect responses. Next, count the total number of items on which at least one perseverative response occurred. (*Caution:* Do not count multiple perseverations for an item, but only the number of items that elicited one or more perseverations.) Perseverations are defined as part/whole recurrent productions of any previously produced response, whether or not they are self-corrected. More specifically, perseveration (of the recurrent type) can be divided into two groups:

    a. **Semantic perseveration,** the **delayed** recurrence of a whole word that is a previously produced response that may or may not be related to the target category.

        Examples: shoulder → "shoulder"
        ankle → "ankle"
        *wrist → "shoulder"
        7 → "7"
        15 → "15"
        700 → "700"
        1936 → "36" . . . "1936"
        *42 → "7"

        *items eliciting perseveration

    b. **Phonemic carryover,** the **immediate or delayed** recurrence of a part word or phoneme(s).

        Examples: chair → "ready"
        *key → "rik"
        *glove → "ratio"
        *feather → "radio"
        *hammock → "radio"
        nose → "nove"

*elbow → "nuvle"
*shoulder → "shuvle"

items eliciting perseveration

2. Divide the number of items that elicited at least one per-severation by 38 (total number of BDAE stimuli). For example, a patient producing perseverative responses for 11 of the 38 items would earn a perseveration rating of 29%. Use this ratio to assign a perseveration severity rating according to the following scale:

   a. Under 5% (minimal perseveration): 1

   b. 5–19% (mild perseveration): 2

   c. 20–49% (moderate perseveration): 3

   d. Above 49% (severe perseveration): 4

   Patients receiving a perseveration severity rating of 3 (moderate) or 4 (severe) can be considered candidates for the TAP program.

C. Preparing for a TAP Session

It is axiomatic that aphasia treatment begins where the patient has the greatest chance of success and proceeds in small incre-ments of difficulty. Before beginning TAP, therefore, it is important to identify the hierarchy of difficulty for the seman-tic categories for each individual patient. For the first session of TAP, the clinician can determine this hierarchy according to the patient's performance on the BDAE. The following pro-cedure is used:

1. Establish a hierarchy of each patient's performance on the BDAE Visual Confrontation Naming subtest by ordering the semantic categories from strongest to weakest. This hierarchy is determined by calculating two ratios:

   a. Divide the number of points earned for each semantic category by the total number of possible points within each category (e.g., Objects = 18 possible points; Geo-metric Forms = 6 possible points). A score of 8/18 on Objects = 44%; a score of 2/6 on Geometric Forms = 33%.

   b. Calculate a perseveration score for each semantic cate-gory by dividing the number of stimulus items that elic-

TABLE 17.1
Hierarchy of Semantic Difficulty for Patient A

% of perseverative responses	Category	% correct responses
(strongest) 1/6 = 17%	Actions	15/18 = 83% (first)
6/6 = 0%	Body parts	6/18 = 33%
1/2 = 50%	Geometric forms	3/6 = 17%
5/6 = 83%	Letters	3/18 = 11%
4/6 = 67%	Colors	2/18 = 0%
4/6 = 67%	Numbers	0/18 = 0%
(weakest) 5/6 = 83%	Objects	0/18 = 0% last

ited at least one perseveration into the total number of stimulus items (e.g., 3 of 6 actions elicited perseveration = 50%).

2. Use these pairs of scores to order the semantic categories from strongest (highest percentage of score points and lowest ratio of perseverations) to weakest (lowest percentage of score points and highest ratio of perseverations). This hierarchy of difficulty determines the order of presentation of semantic categories for TAP, proceeding from the easiest to the most difficult, as in the example of Patient A (see Table 17.1).

After the first TAP session, the order of difficulty and presentation for the next session is based on the patient's response to the TAP items during the first session. This hierarchy is established by analyzing the patient's response to each session according to the prescribed TAP scoring system (detailed later in section E).

Before beginning the TAP program, the clinician must prepare the 38 stimulus items. Where possible, real items (or realistic substitutes) should be used for the earlier sessions, but pictured representations should be prepared for all items. All patients are administered the same stimuli to begin, but sometimes substitutions must be made for items that prove too difficult (e.g., numbers and letters). In such cases the clinician should introduce items that are more personalized, such as the patient's date of birth, age, or initials.

D. General and Specific Strategies

The TAP program employs several general strategies that are used with all patients and 11 specific strategies or cues that are used according to the individual patient's naming performance and response to these cues. The general strategies proceed as follows:

1. Begin the initial session by explaining the TAP program to the patient. Discuss why he or she is in this particular program (i.e., that he tends to say words he said before even when he doesn't mean to, that he seems to get "stuck" on some words). Explain that this is called *perseveration* (write the word down) and that the TAP program is designed to help with this problem. Give the patient examples of his or her perseveration, not only at this point but throughout the program. For example, "Mrs. M, you're perseverating (or stuck) on that word. You've already said that before and it's not appropriate now. Be careful and try not to say that word again. Either give me a different word, or don't say anything and ask for help." Try to combine humor with forcefulness in pointing out perseverations, so that the patient becomes sensitized to the errors but not frustrated by them or intimidated by the clinician.

2. Clearly establish each new set before offering a new stimulus (i.e., emphasize to the patient that you are going to present either a *new item* or a *different category*). With some patients it may be necessary to "chat" between items and categories or to engage briefly in a nonverbal task such as block design in order to avoid "stuck-in-set" types of perseveration.

3. When a patient is perseverating on a particular word within therapy, it may be effective to (a) tell the patient that he or she keeps saying the same word over and over and that it is not correct for any of the TAP items, (b) write the incorrect, perseverative response on a piece of paper so the patient can see it, and then (c) rip the paper up and leave the pieces in the patient's field of vision as a reminder. Every time the patient begins to say this word again, point to the pieces quickly to help him or her inhibit the response.

4. Always monitor the presentation pace for the stimuli, observing at least 5-second intervals between items.

The 11 specific strategies are used to elicit correct, nonperseverative responses from the patient. Although the list that follows shows these cues ranked from minimal to maximal assistance, they are not necessarily listed in the correct hierarchy of difficulty for a particular patient. Instead, the clinician must determine the best of these strategies, based on the patient's performance during the entire aphasia evaluation and through trial and error. If the patient's response to a particular stimulus is immediately correct, a new item is presented after at least a 5-second delay with a comment such as "Here's a new letter." If the response is incorrect, a cue is given. If the response to the cue is correct, the patient must answer the question, "So what is this?" In the attempt to elicit a correct, nonperseverative response followed by confrontation naming, no more than three specific cues can be used before a new item is presented. The clinician should try to reduce the strength of the cues (e.g., instead of writing out the whole word, present just the first letter). Descriptions of the specific strategies follow:

1. **Time interval (TI).** Impose a 5- or 10-second time interval between presentation of stimulus and patient's verbal response. Help the patient inhibit verbalization during these intervals.

2. **Gestural Cue (GC).** Provide a pantomime associated with the object (e.g., gesture winding or listening to a watch).

3. **Tactile Cue (TC).** Ask the patient to hold or appropriately manipulate the real object (e.g., put the watch on his or her wrist).

4. **Drawing (D).** Begin to draw a picture of the item while the patient looks on, asking him or her to tell you what it is as soon as he or she recognizes it. If this is not successful, then ask the patient to draw the item.

5. **Descriptive Sentence (DS).** Provide a descriptive sentence for the stimulus (e.g., "You use this to tell time").

6. **Sentence Completion (SC).** Provide an open-ended sentence that might elicit the target word (e.g., "You tell time with your _____ ").

7. **Graphic Cue (GC).** Write the first letter or two of the word and ask the patient to identify it, or ask the patient to complete the writing and then read it aloud.

8. **Phonemic Cue (PhC).** Provide the initial phoneme of the target word (e.g., "This is a w____").

9. **Oral Reading (OR).** Write the entire target word and ask the patient to read it aloud.

10. **Repetition (R).** Say the word for the patient and ask him or her to repeat it.

11. **Unison Speech or Singing (US).** Ask the patient to say or sing the word with you (e.g., "Say this word with me—a *watch*").

E. The TAP Scoring System

Two aspects of the patient's performance are measured in the TAP program: (a) the ability to name correctly without or with cues, and (b) the incidence of perseverative responses made while attempting to name the TAP item. These two measures are used to chart progress, to determine the order of presentation for the next session, and to determine the effectiveness of specific cues. Score sheets are used to record the performance for each session. The Naming score for each item is computed thusly:

8 = Correctly named without a cue

7 = Self-corrected without a cue

6 = Correctly named with one cue

5 = Self-corrected with one cue

4 = Correctly named with two cues

3 = Self-corrected with two cues

2 = Correctly named after three cues

1 = Self-corrected with three cues

0 = Could not name even after three cues

Whereas in naming the higher the score, the better the performance, when scoring perseveration the opposite is true. The higher the Perseveration score, the poorer the performance. The Perseveration score for each item is computed as follows:

0 = No perseveration

1 = Self-corrected perseveration on first perseveration of the item

2 = Non-corrected perseveration(s) on first perseveration of the item

3 = Self-corrected perseveration with first cue

4 = Non-corrected perseveration(s) with first cue

5 = Self-corrected perseveration(s) with second cue

6 = Non-corrected perseveration(s) with third cue

7 = Self-corrected perseveration(s) with third cue

8 = Non-corrected perseveration(s) with third cue

These two scores (Naming and Perseveration) are recorded on two charts, one for general progress and one for specific performance. The general progress goal is to see the Naming score climb while the Perseveration score declines. If this does not occur, then the program may be inappropriate for a particular patient. The purpose of the specific performance chart is to note the order of difficulty for each item and semantic category for each session. These scores are used to (a) replace items that are too difficult, and (b) establish the order of presentation (easiest to hardest) for the next session.

F. Measuring the Effects of TAP

As just mentioned, the within-treatment goal of TAP is for the patient to show an increase in naming and decrease in perseveration from one session to the next. If this trend is not seen over five sessions, then one should reevaluate the appropriateness of this method. Even if session-by-session progress is noted, every 10 sessions an independent measure of response should be administered. Because TAP is aimed at reducing perseveration and improving naming performance, the clinician may use the Confrontation Naming subtest of the BDAE as the independent measure. The same procedure described previously under candidacy selection (section B) is used for measuring generalization or response to TAP. At the same time one should readminister the "Cookie Theft" picture description task at 10-session intervals as a measure of narrative language skills.

References and Suggested Readings

Albert, M.L., & Sandson, J. (1986). Perseveration in aphasia. *Cortex, 22,* 103–115.

Emery, P., & Helm-Estabrooks, N. (1989). The role of perseveration in confrontation naming performance. In T. Prescott (Ed.)., *Proceedings of the Conference of Clinical Aphasiology* (pp. 271–280). Austin, TX: PRO-ED.

Helm-Estabrooks, N., Emery, P., & Albert, M.L. (1987). Treatment of Aphasic Perseveration (TAP) program. *Archives of Neurology, 44,* 1253–1255.

Sandson, J., & Albert, M.L. (1984). Varieties of perseveration. *Neuropsychologia, 22,* 715–732.

Appendix: TAP Stimuli

Objects	Actions	Colors
money	crying	green
gun	painting	black
shoe	eating	yellow
egg	fighting	white
house	whistling	gold
watch	laughing	orange

Letters	Numbers	Body Parts
B	1	hand
I	6	back
V	20	teeth
E	500	arm
D	3000	foot
O	1945	eye

Geometric Forms

cross

heart

18 Treatment for Wernicke's Aphasia

As was detailed in chapter 8, most aphasic individuals, if tested extensively, can be shown to have at least mild impairment of auditory comprehension. Conversely, virtually no aphasic patient is without the ability to process some language information presented auditorily. This latter point is supported by the finding that 92% of globally and severely aphasic patients tested by the *Boston Assessment of Severe Aphasia* responded correctly to the oral command "Close your eyes." One possible explanation for this finding can be traced to Geschwind (1975), who noted that the command to close one's eyes is carried out by the more intact extrapyramidal motor system rather than by the damaged pyramidal motor system. In addition, commands such as "Close your eyes" are highly familiar, occurring in many natural settings, unlike commands such as "Point to the ceiling." This is not to say that clinicians should limit exploration to naturalistic commands when examining auditory comprehension; a thorough examination will include a wide variety of material in order to identify impaired skills in mildly impaired patients.

After delineating the nature of the auditory comprehension deficit in a particular patient, the clinician then must decide whether the existing deficits significantly interfere with the patient's daily life. If the answer to this question is "yes," then one must consider a course of therapeutic intervention. If it is "no," then concentration instead should shift to other defective skills that do affect communicative interchange. For example, although some individuals with Broca's aphasia have some degree of difficulty understanding complex syntactic constructions, the clinician might rightfully decide that it is more important to concentrate on verbal output problems. In Broca's aphasia, after all, it is the difficulty in verbal expression that contributes most significantly to the breakdown in communication. In contrast, the patient with Wernicke's aphasia often is notably handicapped by an inability to process auditory material, although his or her paraphasic, empty speech output may contribute equally to the communication problem.

The treatment of Wernicke's aphasia is particularly challenging. In 1948 Neilson and his colleagues pointed out that if taught to read, write, and do arithmetic, the sensory (Wernicke's) aphasic patient would automatically relearn spoken language. This observation was tested, in part, in a case study by Ulatowska and Richardson (1974). As their patient had failed to show significant response to "traditional techniques" (e.g., pointing to objects and pictures on command), these researchers instituted a deblocking program that used written stimuli as a stable representation for reinforcing auditory stimuli. (It should be noted that there is a distinct group of Wernicke's aphasic patients whose reading comprehension is significantly superior to their auditory comprehension, and Ulatowska and Richardson's patient was among this group.) The deblocking program included the following tasks: (a) sequencing written words into sentences, (b) matching written phrases to pictures, (c) pointing to these phrases on oral command, (d) pointing to individual words in the phrases, (e) pointing to pictures associated with the phrases, (f) answering questions about the phrases, and (g) providing oral descriptions of the pictures. Improvement was seen in auditory and reading comprehension and in verbal expression.

Perhaps the most startling evidence that auditory comprehension skills may be deblocked through a different modality is found in the 1982 study of Visual Action Therapy (see chapter 12). In VAT no spoken or written words are used in training patients to produce representational gestures for absent objects. Despite this fact, eight globally aphasic subjects treated with VAT improved significantly in auditory processing skills as measured by the *Porch Index of Communicative Ability*.

Improved auditory comprehension is also a common "side effect" of Melodic Intonation Therapy, a method that employs verbal repetition (see chapter 15). In an unpublished study of the generalized effects of MIT (described in Helm-Estabrooks, 1983), auditory comprehension for *Boston Diagnostic Aphasia Examination* (BDAE) complex ideational material (sentences and paragraphs) was found to improve significantly in a group of 22 nonfluent patients treated with MIT.

Improvement of auditory comprehension skills as a result of improved ability to repeat words and phrases may be explained by a process Jones and Wepman (1961) called **reauditorization**: the transmission of aurally received stimuli into verbal responses. These investigators conducted a factor analysis of the components of language performance in aphasia and found a positive relationship between oral repetition ability and the ability to point to visual stimuli named by the examiner. Clinically, one observes that some patients with Wernicke's aphasia may point correctly to items on the BDAE Word Discrimination subtest only after they have spontaneously repeated the stimulus words correctly. This same effect does not appear in patients with transcortical sensory aphasia, who may repeat single words flawlessly without a sense of the meaning. Luria (1980) refers to this latter phenomenon as the **extinction of word meaning**, or the alienation of the meaning from the acoustic representation of words. He notes that this is a very different auditory problem than that seen in lesions of the cortical areas, including Wernicke's area, responsible for analyzing auditory stimuli.

In the past few years Helm-Estabrooks and Fitzpatrick have developed a treatment approach to Wernicke's aphasia based on the evidence that ability to repeat orally presented stimuli may be linked to the ability to process or understand these stimuli. In a manner similar to Ulatowska and Richardson (1974), this method (called Treatment for Wernicke's Aphasia, or TWA) uses written stimuli as the initial stable representation of the stimulus words. TWA progresses, however, from reading comprehension, to oral reading, to oral repetition, and then to auditory comprehension alone. Although no formal study of this aphasia program has been undertaken, Helm-Estabrooks and Fitzpatrick have used it to treat several individuals with Wernicke's aphasia with good results.

A. The Treatment for Wernicke's Aphasia (TWA) Program

Treatment for Wernicke's Aphasia (TWA) begins by using the more intact modality of reading comprehension to stimulate oral reading. Words that are orally read correctly then are presented verbally for repetition and finally for auditory comprehension via a picture pointing task. The initial choice of stimuli is determined by the individual's performance on an aphasia test; that is, the initial stimuli are those that the patient can read aloud correctly. Subsequent stimuli are added in a manner similar to that used in Voluntary Control of Involuntary Utterances (see chapter 14) until the patient is capable of handling minimal pair words (i.e., those differing by only one phoneme).

B. Candidacy for the TWA Program

As its name implies, the Treatment for Wernicke's Aphasia is a syndrome-specific treatment approach. (The reader is referred to chapter 3 for differential diagnosis of Wernicke's aphasia.) Furthermore, TWA is appropriate only for moderate to severe Wernicke's aphasia patients who have difficulty processing single words through the auditory modality. In addition to these characteristics, TWA candidates must demonstrate relatively good ability to understand written stimuli at the single-word level (as demonstrated by picture-to-word matching skills) and some ability to correctly read picturable single words aloud. If oral reading is poor on a formal test such as the BDAE, then the patient should be asked to read aloud words with high emotional valence (e.g., *blood, gun*). In summary, good candidates for TWA will display the following characteristics:

1. A diagnosis of severe Wernicke's aphasia (i.e., fluent, paraphasic output, with poor auditory comprehension skills and poor oral repetition skills); more specifically,

   a. an overall Auditory Comprehension score no greater than the 40th percentile on the BDAE, with single-word discrimination no greater than the 45th percentile, and
   b. an overall BDAE Repetition score no greater than the 30th percentile.

2. Relatively preserved single-word reading comprehension skills, as evidenced by a score at or above the 50th percentile on the BDAE subtest of Word-Picture Matching.

3. Some ability to read single, picturable words aloud. Words that may be used to test this ability include the following:

beer	candy	eat	gun	fire
heart	money	smoke	police	school
booze	priest	fight	home	pills

Note: These words, as well as those presented in TWA, are always presented in lowercase so that the configuration of ascenders and descenders is preserved. In fact, the reader will note that all of the words just listed are configural, a variable that often enhances the reading performances of aphasic patients. Similarly, words such as *moon* that have double letters are often read aloud correctly.

C. Selection of Stimuli

The first step in implementing TWA is to establish a corpus of words (printed in lowercase) that the patient can (a) match with their pictorial representation and (b) read aloud correctly. Words other than those just listed in the previous section may be obtained from the individual patient's performance on a formal test. For example, Mr. S matched the BDAE word *chair* to the picture of a chair, and during the Word Reading subtest he also was able to read this word aloud. He did not, however, repeat "chair" correctly during the Word Repetition subtest, nor did he point to the picture of a chair in the Auditory Word Discrimination subtest. The word *chair,* therefore, was added to his initial TWA list for deblocking through reading, repetition, and reauditorization. The clinician may obtain additional stimuli by presenting other high-probability, high-emotion words, or even low-probability words with a unique configuration (e.g., *zoo*). From session to session the word list should expand, as the patient's own real word errors are used in a manner similar to Voluntary Control of Involuntary Utterances. When the patient has demonstrated the ability to recognize about 100 words through the auditory modality by pointing to pictures on command, picturable minimal pairs should be slowly introduced. The following are examples of appropriate minimal pairs:

mat/hat	beer/bear	tile/dial
seat/seed	pin/pill	top/mop

This list can be expanded as the patient demonstrates that he or she can reliably identify pairs of stimuli (e.g., *cat, fat, rat, vat, bat*).

D. Presentation of Stimuli

Four steps comprise the hierarchically organized TWA format. If the patient fails to perform any step with a particular stimulus, then the nature of the incorrect response is noted, that item is set aside for a future trial, and a new stimulus word is introduced at step 1. The TWA tasks proceed in the following order:

1. Matching a printed, lowercase word to its pictorial representation.

2. Reading this word aloud.

3. Repeating this word as presented by the clinician without the presence of the printed stimulus.

4. Correctly selecting the pictorial representation of this word from a group of eight upon hearing the word spoken by the clinician (again without benefit of the printed stimulus).

The clinician should transcribe all incorrect verbal responses and note all incorrect picture choices. Incorrect verbal responses that are real words are used as stimuli in subsequent sessions.

E. Charting Progress in TWA

A score sheet with space for listing the target words and the response to each step will help chart progress in TWA. After an item has been identified successfully at step 4 over two successive sessions, it is dropped from the list and new items are added. If the method is appropriate for a particular patient, after the third session the master list of correctly identified words will begin to expand and the session-to-session list will start to change. If this does not occur after five sessions, then either the program may need modification or another approach may need to be considered. In any case, the clinician should reevaluate the target behavior (auditory comprehension) after 12 sessions to measure the effects of treatment.

References and Selected Readings

Geschwind, N. (1975). The apraxias: Neural mechanisms of learned movement. *American Scientist, 63,* 188–195.

Helm-Estabrooks, N. (1983). Exploiting the right hemisphere for language rehabilitation: Melodic Intonation Therapy. In E. Perecman (Ed.), *Cognitive processing in the right hemisphere* (pp. 229–240). New York: Academic Press.

Jones, L.V., & Wepman, J.M. (1961). Dimensions of language performance in aphasia. *Journal of Speech and Hearing Research, 4,* 220–232.

Luria, A.R. (1980). *Higher cortical functions in man* (2nd ed.). New York: Basic Books.

Neilson, J.M., Schutz, D.H., Corbin, M.L., & Crittsinger, B. (1948). The treatment of traumatic aphasia of WWII at Birmingham General VA Hospital, Van Nuys, California. *Military Surgery, 10,* 351–364.

Ulatowska, H.R., & Richardson, S.M. (1974). A longitudinal study of an adult with aphasia: Considerations for research and therapy. *Brain and Language, 1,* 151–166.

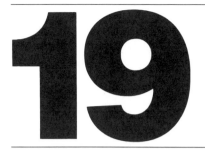

Pharmacotherapy for Aphasia

Neurotransmitters are chemical substances that allow (electrochemical) messages to be sent from one nerve cell to another. Among the better known neurotransmitters are **dopamine, norepinephrine, serotonin,** and **acetylcholine**. When dopamine is reduced in the brain, as in Parkinson's disease, the result is called a **dopaminergic deficiency**. When norepinephrine (also called **noradrenalin**) is low in the brain, the term is **adrenergic deficiency**, and when acetycholine is reduced, as in Alzheimer's disease, the patient has a **cholinergic deficiency**.

Speech-language pathologists may be familiar with the use of dopamine or dopaminergic agents to treat Parkinson's disease. This condition incurs a slowing of all movements and a peculiar speech disorder, which is characterized by an impairment in the ability to initiate speech, followed by a rapid, low-pitched, hypophonic, stuttering-like **palilalia** (i.e., rapid repetition of one's own words and phrases). Treatment with dopamine in such cases may allow the patient to initiate speech and other movements, increase the speed of response, and reduce palilalia.

Neuroscientists are actively involved in an intensive search for the many other neurotransmitters that facilitate transmission of nerve impulses. Dozens of likely candidates have been discovered, including **neuropeptides** such as enkephalin, endorphin, and somatostatin, and a variety of **amino acids**, such as gamma-amino butyric acid, or GABA. Within the past decade there has been an increase in the number of researchers who are using neurotransmitters and other chemical agents to treat signs of cognitive impairment due to cerebral dysfunction. The best known, but as yet unsuccessful, experiments are those attempting to improve the memory disorder of Alzheimer's disease by treatment with cholinergic agents. Surprisingly, there has been little systematic investigation of neurotransmitters that may be helpful in the treatment of aphasia. Two approaches to pharmacotherapy for aphasia may be considered. The first addresses therapy for the neurobehavioral or psychiatric complications of aphasia; the second, therapy for specific linguistic deficits.

I. Pharmacotherapy for Psychiatric Complications of Brain Damage

Although several of the neurobehavioral phenomena that may accompany aphasic syndromes (described in chapter 20) may be amenable to pharmacotherapy, the clinician should not consider treating these disorders phamacologically as a first resort. A calm, comforting, reassuring, confident, and supportive attitude on the part of the therapist can significantly affect how successfully persons with aphasia overcome their shock, disappointment, fear, anger, frustration, and loneliness. We rarely, if ever, resort to chemical agents for management of these emotional reactions that we consider to be normal reactions in adjusting to the reality of aphasia.

Many persons with aphasia eventually will adapt to their loss. Some, however, have greater difficulty with depression than others, despite all the support offered by a clinician or by the family. A speech-language pathologist should feel free to consult frequently with a psychologist, psychiatrist, or behavioral neurologist. Reactive depression can be managed by several treatment modalities, and it may be best to ask a physician to intervene.

Lesions in the left frontal lobe that produce severe nonfluent aphasia commonly produce a major depressive disorder as well. Clinical experience and experimental evidence suggest that this syndrome of depression may be related to lesion site and may be different from the reactive depression common to all individuals who have suffered a serious loss. The **frontal-lobe depression syndrome** may overwhelm the patient's ability to accept or respond to language therapy and may persist for weeks or months. In such cases one might consider treating the patient with a **tricyclic antidepressant agent**—imipramine or a related substance. Often this treatment will lift the depression and facilitate aphasia therapy.

A similar lesion, perhaps located somewhat more anteriorly, can produce a **catastrophic reaction** (described in chapter 20). Here, again, some success may be achieved by treating this disorder with tricyclic antidepressant agents. More recently, we have turned to **beta-blocking agents**, such as propanolol, instead of tricyclic antidepressants for the treatment of catastrophic reaction. When they work, which is certainly not in all cases, beta-blocking agents have the advantage of taking effect more rapidly.

Severe, extreme **anxiety or agitation** may be treated with the usual **anxiolytic or psychotropic agents** in current use. As stated previously, however, most people with aphasia will not need these drugs and will respond to the sensitive, supportive care of a sympathetic therapist.

II. Pharmacotherapy for Specific Language Disorders

In ancient times wine, berries, roots, herbs, and nuts, especially cashews, were used as ingestible agents for the treatment of aphasia. Similar efforts in modern times have included chemical agents such as caffeine, aspirin, sodium amytal, and amphetamine. At the time of this writing, however, no phamacologic agent has yet proven effective for the treatment of aphasia in any systematic, controlled, experimental research. A strong, intellectually appealing argument can be made, however, that selected features of aphasia may result from disruption of specific neurotransmitter systems. If this were the case, then replacement of these neurotransmitters might influence recovery from aphasia when administered in conjunction with ongoing language therapy.

When brain tissue is injured, recovery follows a characteristic pattern. Initially, there is local edema and distant suppression of metabolic activity in regions connected with the area of destruction, called **diaschisis**. At the site of the lesion, recovery results from resorption of edema and development of collateral circulation, a process taking several weeks. Recovery from diaschisis may take even longer, as cells that were dysfunctional, but not dead, slowly return to normal metabolic activity.

Denervation supersensitivity develops rapidly. This is a phenomenon in which cells previously dependent on neurons that are now destroyed become supersensitive to neurotransmitters and do not function normally. Recovery from denervation supersensitivity may take months, and may potentially be susceptible to pharmacologic manipulation.

Two additional neurobiologic phenomena also may be considered as potentially subject to pharmacologic treatment: **sprouting** and **latent synapses**. Sprouting of damaged nerve cells is a spontaneous form of recovery. When an axon is damaged, the next neuron in the chain, previously dependent on the damaged axon, becomes supersensitive. Sprouting from adjacent undamaged axons may reestablish disrupted neural connections and may eliminate supersensitivity. Chemical agents may facilitate sprouting.

Latent synapses are silent, underused pathways in the brain that may be inhibited in the normal state by more dominant pathways.

If the dominant pathways are destroyed, the latent synapses may be activated rapidly. Pharmacologic agents can stimulate latent synapses.

The foregoing review suggests several possible ways in which chemical agents could be used to improve behavioral function. We recently explored this approach, focusing on the problem of speech fluency. The decision was made to target selected aphasic symptoms rather than entire aphasic syndromes, and we studied the clinical problems of hesitancy and impaired initiation of speech in transcortical motor aphasia.

The clinical rationale for looking at impaired speech initiation was that Parkinson's disease has features of hesitancy and impaired initiation of movement and responds to dopamine agonists. The theoretical rationale was that mid-brain dopaminergic systems project to medial frontal regions and might be disrupted by medial frontal lesions causing transcortical motor aphasia. Finally, the aphasiological rationale was that hesitancy and impaired initiation of speech are features of transcortical motor aphasia. Thus, we hypothesized that (a) medial frontal lesions could disrupt mesocortical dopaminergic pathways, producing the impaired initiation of speech seen in transcortical motor aphasia, and that (b) this specific aphasia disability might be responsive to pharmacotherapy with the dopaminergic agent bromocriptine.

A handful of patients have now been treated in this way. The first patient showed moderately good results, with improved ability to initiate speech, reduced latency of response, decreased hesitancies, and decreased paraphasias. Other patients have had mixed response to bromocriptine therapy, however. Therefore, it would be inappropriate to claim at this time that any medication has been proven to ameliorate symptoms of aphasia, and likewise it would be unwise and potentially harmful to hold out false hope. Nevertheless, the scientific rationale for continuing to investigate the possibilities of pharmacotherapy of aphasia is sound.

Selected Readings

Albert, M.L., Bachman, D., Morgan, A., & Helm-Estabrooks, N. (1988). Pharmacotherapy of aphasia. *Neurology, 38,* 877–879.

Beckman, A. (1982). *The neural basis of behavior.* New York: Spectrum.

Fleet, W., Watson, R., Valenstein, E., & Heilman, K. (1986). Dopamine agonist therapy for neglect in humans. *Neurology, 36*(Suppl. 1), 347.

Kandel, E., & Schwartz, J. (1981). *Principles of neural science*. New York: Elsevier/North Holland.

Moore, R. (1982). Catecholamine neuron systems in the brain. *Annals of Neurology, 12,* 321–327.

Schiffer, R., Herndon, R., & Rudick, R. (1985). Treatment of pathologic laughing and weeping with amitriptylene. *New England Journal of Medicine, 312,* 1480–1482.

Section Five

**Impact of Aphasia on
the Patient and Family**

20 Psychological and Neuropsychiatric Aspects of Aphasia

The psychological aspects of aphasia can be considered from two points of view. First, brain lesions that produce language impairments also may induce other behavioral changes linked specifically to the site of the lesion. These changes are termed the **neurobehavioral aspects** of aphasia. Second, one can look at the **emotional reactions** that individuals experience with regard to their sudden loss of language. Any attempt to treat a person with aphasia must take into account both of these psychological responses—one neurobehavioral, the other reactive—because both can occur, and each can influence the other.

Table 20.1 presents a brief and schematic clinical guide to the neurobehavioral correlates of aphasia. The clinician must be mindful, however, of cases where the "rules" do not apply. Certainly not all aphasics develop an associated brain lesion–induced emotional syndrome. Additionally, exceptions to the correlations summarized in Table 20.1 may occur. For example, one may see patients with Wernicke's aphasia who have severe depression, as opposed to the more common pattern of unawareness, agitation, and paranoia, thus belying the often repeated claim that auditory comprehension must be reasonably intact for a true depression to develop. Nonetheless, patterns summarized in Table 20.1 are not unusual.

TABLE 20.1
Neurobehavioral Correlates of Aphasia

Sign/symptom	Aphasia type	Lesion localization
Denial/catastrophic reaction	Broca's, global	Frontal
Depression	Broca's, global	Frontal (cortical or subcortical)
Unawareness	Wernicke's	Posterior temporal
Agitation (with or without paranoia)	Word deafness, Wernicke's	Temporal
Hypomania (rare)	Anomia	Parietal (angular gyrus)

I. Neuropsychiatric Aspects of Aphasia

Denial of illness is a common phenomenon following brain damage and probably has different underlying mechanisms depending on lesion localization. Usually, denial of illness is discussed in relation to right-hemispheric lesions. However, there are forms that follow left-hemispheric, aphasia-producing lesions. Three varieties of denial may be associated with aphasia: **catastrophic reaction**, **indifference**, and **unawareness**.

The **catastrophic reaction**, which has been called a disturbance in the patient's ability to maintain biologic homeostasis, can be considered a form of massive denial. Clinically, one may see a severe form of rejection reaction following left frontal lobe damage with resulting global or Broca's aphasia. The patient switches suddenly, and often violently, into a state of intense negativity. The high degree of correlation with this particular lesion localization and the stereotypic pattern of response strongly suggest that this behavior is not completely within the realm of voluntary control. The highly complex nature of the behavior, however, suggests that some degree of volition may play a role. Ordinarily, catastrophic reactions, treated with patience, sympathy, and understanding, will dissipate within a few days. However, one may see globally aphasic patients with a catastrophic reaction lasting several months. In such cases the patient exhibits easy frustration and may withdraw from all activities, refuse to go to therapy, refuse to take medicines, and so forth. Occasionally such patients may benefit from pharmacotherapy, either with tricyclic antidepressants or with beta-adrenergic blocking agents.

An **indifference reaction** may develop if the left frontal lobe lesion extends sufficiently forward into the prefrontal, especially dorsolateral, region. Such responses are not common with aphasia due to stroke but are often seen with aphasia caused by traumatic brain injury. The patient seems to have a bland disregard for the disorder affecting his or her ability to communicate and shows no apparent interest in the efforts being made by friends, family, and medical staff. With complete equanimity such a patient may, for example, urinate on himself in his wheelchair and ignore his wetness, sitting there in a puddle until someone comes by to clean him up. In this clinical condition, the patient is aware of the problem (and therefore does not have an unawareness syndrome) but is calmly indifferent, thereby distinguishing him- or herself from the patient with a catastrophic reaction.

Unawareness of the deficit is another form of denial and is linked to the posterior temporal lobe lesions that may produce Wernicke's aphasia. Unlike the indifference reaction, in which the patient though aware seems not to be bothered by distressing events, these patients do not seem to know that anything is wrong. Such a patient may act as if he were carrying on a perfectly normal conversation, even though he doesn't comprehend what is being said to him (because of his auditory comprehension deficit) and his listener doesn't understand what he is saying (because of his neologistic jargon).

Unawareness of an aphasic deficit in someone who cannot understand spoken language (as in word deafness) or who cannot understand that his or her verbal production may be neologistic and incomprehensible (as in Wernicke's aphasia) may lead to awkward, uncomfortable social interactions. In such situations patients can become **agitated** and occasionally **difficult to control**. In patients recovering from severe Wernicke's aphasia or word deafness, **suspiciousness** and even frank **paranoia** may emerge. As impairments of auditory acuity in nonaphasics may be a cause of paranoid behavior, it is possible that the impairments of auditory-system functioning in Wernicke's aphasia or word deafness may contribute to paranoia. Failure to understand speech may lead patients to believe that others are talking about them in a special code. Fully developed paranoid psychoses, however, are not common in aphasia.

Depression, indistinguishable from Major Depressive Disorder (in standard psychiatric terminology), has been linked reliably to strokes in the left frontal region, either cortical or subcortical. Lesions in the same regions that cause depression also can produce nonfluent aphasic syndromes. Thus, probably by virtue of overlapping anatomical bases, nonfluent aphasia and depression commonly are seen together. We hypothesize that the same neurobiological mechanisms that underlie depression due to left frontal damage also may be at the root of catastrophic reactions. Indeed, it is likely that depression and catastrophic reaction, if they are not identical, have overlapping clinical and neurobiological features. Clinicians may be concerned about the effects of depression or catastrophic reaction in response to language therapy. In such cases it is possible that pharmacological treatment of the depression with antidepressant medication might facilitate response to aphasia therapy, although this possibility has not been studied systematically.

The association of **hypomania** and anomic aphasia, which occasionally is observed, has received little attention in the scientific literature. Such patients seem excited, ebullient, and hyperfluent. Like patients in the hypomanic phase of Bipolar Affective Disorder, verbal output is circumstantial and ideas do not always flow smoothly from one to another. Probably the lack of control over semantic aspects of communication underlies much of the behavior of the anomic aphasic, but the hyperfluency and excitability remain to be explained.

It should be noted, of course, that not all emotional reactions following brain damage are necessarily negative. For example, we have noticed during aphasia rounds how "nice" our patients with conduction aphasia seem to be. This observation may be nothing more than chance; it may also be that the conduction aphasics stand out because other aphasics in our population more often have associated psychiatric symptoms. However, an alternative explanation is that the lesion producing conduction aphasia may be associated with positive emotional and personality changes.

II. Psychosocial Aspects of Aphasia

The psychosocial/emotional aspects of aphasia are, perhaps, even more disabling than neurobehavioral aspects. Due to the loss of language, an aphasic person's fundamental link with other human beings and with his or her own sense of personhood is altered profoundly. With the breaking of the communication link, a cascade of social disturbances descends on the person with aphasia.

Social isolation and **loneliness** develop rapidly. Often unable to work, the aphasic must withdraw from daily contacts with coworkers. Many people feel uncomfortable trying to communicate with aphasic acquaintances; thus, friends and neighbors tend to distance themselves. Even within the family, anger and frustration on the part of the spouse and children will further isolate the person with aphasia. In our long-term aphasia follow-up study, a sense of loneliness and isolation and a feeling of rejection were common complaints of aphasic patients.

Elizabeth Kübler-Ross has spoken of the steps of psychological reaction to a profound loss or devastating disease. **Denial** (unrelated to focal lesions) is a key step in this process for both the patient and his or her family. With this in mind, the clinician should always try to be sensitive to the possibility of neurologically induced *and* situationally induced (or reactive) denial in the patient, in addition to denial in the patient's family as well.

Anger is another step in the process that leads ultimately to acceptance, according to Kübler-Ross. The patient with aphasia will evidence signs of anger and frustration not only because of the personal loss but also because of society's reaction. "Stupid," "mentally retarded," "crazy," and "drunk" are some of the labels routinely attached to aphasic persons by a general public ignorant of the true nature of the disorder.

Although obvious, it seems important to state nonetheless that clinicians must regard their patients as whole human beings and not focus narrowly on the language disorder to the exclusion of the entirety of personhood. The therapist should creatively help the patient with aphasia regain language function to the extent possible, but at the same time effort should be made toward helping the patient accommodate to the reality of impaired function—learning to live with and compensate for deficits.

Equally dramatic as the effects of aphasia on the patient are the changes that occur in his or her family life. The aphasic spouse and parent can no longer fulfill his or her role within the family. From the position of independent economic provider or household keeper, the aphasic person suddenly falls to a level of dependency. The family may have to cope with a sudden and unexpected decrease in income; the patient's spouse faces full responsibility where formerly family burdens were halved and shared. Dramatic alterations in sexual relations are a common consequence of aphasia. Changes in the small details of everyday life often become the most burdensome and poignant. The wife of a severely aphasic patient told us that one of the hardest parts of living alone with him was that suddenly there was no one to talk with—that is, to have real discussions with—at mealtimes. Conversations became one-sided; her husband could no longer offer advice or tell little jokes, as he used to.

For children, the change in image of the now-aphasic parent can be frightening and confusing. Children may begin to "act out," which only compounds the problem. Anger, pain, fear, anxiety, bitterness, and frustration are the anticipated and usual result of aphasia within a family. For many families, the strain is beyond their ability to cope, and divorce or separation may result.

Often whoever tells the aphasic patient "You have aphasia" does not go on to explain what that means. We have frequently cared for aphasic persons and their families who have told us that no one had previously explained what had happened in the brain and why the aphasic person was having problems with language—not the physician, not the aphasia therapist, no one. Most lay people have never heard about aphasia before it happens to them, and they cannot figure it out by themselves.

The clinician must be sensitive to issues of neurobehavioral and psychosocial concern and be prepared to intervene, either directly or by means of appropriate consultation. It is not enough just to apply a specific aphasia therapy technique. The goal of treatment includes helping the patient cope with residual deficits and helping patient and family learn to relate to each other with a new form of communication.

Selected Readings

Benson, D.F. (1973). Psychiatric aspects of aphasia. *British Journal of Psychiatry, 123,* 555–566.

Friedman, M.H. (1961). On the nature of regression in aphasia. *Archives of General Psychiatry, 5,* 60–64.

Gainotti, G. (1972). Emotional behavior and hemispheric side of lesion. *Cortex, 8,* 41–55.

Goldstein, K. (1942). *After effects of brain injuries in war.* New York: Grune & Stratton.

Heilman, K., & Valenstein, E. (1985). *Clinical neuropsychology* (2nd ed.). New York: Oxford University Press.

Horenstein, S. (1970). Effects of cerebrovascular disease on personality and emotionality. In A.L. Benton (Ed.). *Behavioral change in cerebrovascular disease.* New York: Harber.

Sarno, J. (1983). *Understanding aphasia: A guide for family and friends.* New York: New York University Medical Center, Institute of Rehabilitation Medicine.

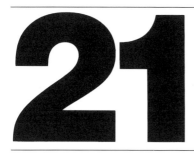

Legal and Social Aspects of Aphasia

Approximately 1 million people have aphasia in the United States today. Although this figure exceeds the number of those who have Parkinson's disease (about 600,000) or muscular dystrophy (about 40,000), aphasia still is relatively unknown and poorly understood as compared to Parkinson's disease or muscular dystrophy. Why is it that aphasia, which causes such devastation for so many people, is so little known? Perhaps because the person with aphasia cannot speak out, and the sudden, dramatic changes in family life are so frightening and isolating, no concerted group effort has been made on behalf of the person with aphasia and his or her family.

This relative lack of societal awareness and support is beginning to change, however, with lawyers, professional groups, and families of persons with aphasia paying more attention to the legal and social aspects of aphasia. Sarno (1986) has suggested that factors that have contributed to the awakening of interest in aphasia may include the emergence of speech pathology as a health profession, the rapid development of the field of rehabilitation medicine, and society's increased expectations from medicine in this age of technology.

Increased attention to ethical issues in an era of increasing financial constraint also may be a contributing factor. Who should receive care, if not everyone can receive it, and who should pay? Questions such as these have led the Hastings Center, an institution concerned with biomedical ethics, to embark on a study of ethical issues in rehabilitation medicine. This 2-year study was designed to answer such ethical questions as when should treatment be initiated and stopped, how should patients be selected for treatment, what are the duties of families, and how should resources be allocated. Aphasia is being addressed in this study along with other aspects of rehabilitation medicine.

I. Legal Implications of Aphasia: Competency

One of the principal legal questions raised when someone becomes aphasic is that of competency. Questions of a legal nature may concern the capacity of a person with aphasia to control his or her own financial affairs, to enter into contracts, or to execute a legally binding will. Underlying these legal questions is a neurobehavioral question: What is the relation of aphasia to intelligence?

Neurologists and cognitive scientists have studied this question for at least the past century. The controversy centers on the following opposing views: (a) Intellectual capacity is lost in aphasia, because language is an integral, inseparable component of intelligence, versus (b) intellectual capacity is not lost in aphasia, because language can be understood as a compartmentalized cognitive capacity and its compromise does not impinge on other, compartmentalized cognitive skills (such as analysis of space). One school of thought holds that intelligence is an all-encompassing synthesis of cognitive skills and that people think in words. According to this school, impairment of language results in an overall lowering of cognitive capacity. In contrast, another popular approach to understanding intelligence holds that human intelligent behavior is the result of a loosely coupled association of independent cognitive skills; loss of one cognitive function would not necessarily impair the capacity of the others (see, for example, Gardner, 1983).

One can take a pragmatic approach to the issue of competency in aphasia without having to wait for a definitive answer to the theoretical questions. If someone asks, "Is this aphasic person competent?" the clinician should begin his or her response by asking "Competent for what?" Many persons with aphasia can carry out some complicated tasks of personal economic relevance, but not others. Although some aphasic patients undoubtedly suffer loss of intellectual capacity, others do not seem to. In either event, regardless of the category into which persons with aphasia may fall, experience shows that many of them (perhaps most) are able to express their wishes clearly despite the loss of language.

Many people with aphasia are capable of conducting their financial and legal affairs without any help and have the desire and need to retain as much control over their lives as possible. Others can carry out such business quite adequately, if given appropriate assistance. Still others, however, may need the protection of a legal guardian. Clinical experience proves that one should not automatically declare all patients with aphasia incompetent. Selected cognitive skills may be preserved, while others are lost.

Competency is a legal concept. Courts must decide if individuals can be accused of criminal responsibility, if they have the capacity to stand trial, if they can execute legal documents, and so on. Decisions of competency in this legal sense are based on individuals' capacity to understand the nature and object of proceedings against them and to assist in their own defense. Courts often turn to physicians to help them make such decisions; however, physicians may make decisions about competency that are based on criteria irrelevant to the law. A patient with a moderately severe nonfluent aphasia, for example, might be considered incompetent by some physicians despite good comprehension of spoken language. The operational question thus remains "Competent for what?"

The steps in the process of determining competency include a careful neurologic examination, a detailed evaluation of language, and a thorough testing of neuropsychological capacity. Analysis of the patient's history (what is the patient actually doing at home and in the rest of his or her life?) is necessary, and at times it may be useful either to bring the patient into the hospital for a few days of observation or to go to the patient's home.

The American Bar Association and the American Speech, Hearing, and Language Association have produced a working document called "Legal Aspects of Aphasia" (Sellers, Downey, & Hantman, 1983). This paper identifies legal issues of concern both to lawyers and to persons with aphasia and their families. Also included is a review of how courts have resolved such issues in the past. Of interest is the explicit statement that "aphasia means that the person's ability to communicate is impaired, not that the individual is mentally incompetent."

Of practical interest, the speech-language pathologist (or any clinician working with an aphasic patient) should keep careful, dated notes and observations of what the aphasic patient actually does. Can he or she use money normally, find his or her own way to therapy sessions, drive a car, play checkers? How does he or she express feelings? Are the social rituals of everyday life preserved? Documentation of such skills may be helpful in legal proceedings.

II. Societal Response to Aphasia

As our society ages, our attitudes toward chronic disease are shifting—slowly. The general public appears to be developing a greater acceptance of and willingness to help people with slowly progressive disorders, such as Alzheimer's disease, and disorders that may require years of care, such as traumatic brain injury. Within the past decade, interested and dedicated individuals have founded such organizations as the National Stroke Association, the Alzheimer's Disease and Related Disorders Association, and the National Head Injury Foundation.

Until 1987 there was no national organization in the United States focusing specifically on the person with aphasia and his or her family. Typically aphasia patients are well treated from a medical and rehabilitation point of view during the first few months following the onset of disability, but after that they receive little or no attention, often regressing steadily into isolation and loneliness. In 1987 the National Aphasia Association (NAA) was formed to meet the need of individuals with aphasia and their families for information and support. The association hopes to serve as an advocate for those distressed by aphasia and its consequences.

The NAA is patterned after successful similar European groups, especially in Sweden, Denmark, and Germany. In Sweden, for example, the aphasia association sponsors public education programs on radio and television, professional conferences, and aphasia support groups in the larger cities. The Swedish association also sponsors programs whereby an aphasic person and family can take a vacation together in an underutilized country hotel with full resort activities. During the visit to the hotel, professional clinical personnel are available to re-evaluate the language disorder and make new suggestions for coping with ongoing problems. The focus in these programs is to help bring persons with aphasia out of their social isolation and to develop mutual support groups. At the same time, family members receive support and respite from their daily burdens.

In the final analysis, rehabilitation of the person with aphasia must be concerned with his or her individual humanity. The aphasic patient may be frightened, lonely, or angry. Whether the clinician works with an aphasic individual, a group of aphasic persons, or a national organization designed to help persons with aphasia, he or she must be a personal ally. The aim must be to understand the person with aphasia as a whole person in a whole context. Even if this person has lost something as precious as language, he or she has retained identity as a person. To maximize an aphasic person's total capacity, despite the disability, is the ultimate goal of aphasia therapy.

References and Suggested Readings

ASHA Committee of Language, Subcommittee on Cognition and Language. (1987). The role of speech-language pathologists in the habilitation and rehabilitation of cognitively impaired individuals. *ASHA, 29,* 53–55.

Gardner, H. (1983). *Frames of mind: A theory of multiple intelligences.* New York: Basic Books.

Sarno, M.T. (1981). Recovery and rehabilitation in aphasia. In M.T. Sarno (Ed.), *Acquired aphasia.* New York: Academic Press.

Sarno, M.T. (1986). *The silent minority: The patient with aphasia* (The 1986 Hemphill Lecture). Chicago: Rehabilitation Institute of Chicago.

Sellers, D., Downey, M., & Hantman, R. (1983). *Legal aspects of aphasia.* American Bar Association, Section of Individual Rights and Responsibilities, Committee on the Rights of Persons with Physical Disabilities, Subcommittee on the Communicatively Handicapped.

Glossary

This glossary consists of terms and acronyms that appear in the patient protocols prepared for our weekly aphasia conferences. Terms listed in the index of this manual are defined in the text and thus are not included in this glossary.

I. Terms

Abulia: The inability to motivate oneself to action.

Acalculia: A disorder in the ability to perform arithmetic operations.

Agnosia: Impairment of the ability to comprehend the meaning of a perceived stimulus.

Akinesia: The absence of movement without paralysis.

Akinetic mutism: A neurologic syndrome in which the individual appears awake and alert but fails to move or speak voluntarily.

Alexia: An acquired disorder of reading secondary to brain damage.

Amnesia: Impairment of memory.

Amusia: Impairment in the ability to process music secondary to brain damage.

Anarthria: Absence of speech due to paralysis of the muscles controlling articulation.

Aprosodia: Loss of the melody, stress, and rhythm patterns of speech.

Astereognosia: Inability to recognize objects through the sense of touch.

Astrocytoma: A brain tumor of glia cell origin, ranging in severity of malignancy.

Asymbolia: Loss of the ability to comprehend and manipulate symbols.

Ataxia: Dyscoordination of movement often associated with cerebellar disease.

Atrophy: Shrinkage of cells or tissue.

Aura: Movements or sensations that may precede an epileptic attack.

Basal ganglia: Subcortical gray matter structures, including putamen, globus pallidus, and caudate, that contribute to control of motor behavior.

Bradyphrenia: The slowing of thought processes.

Bradykinesia: The slowing of movement, often associated with Parkinson's disease.

Chorea: Abnormal involuntary movements characterized by rapid, fluctuating jerkiness.

Clonus: Rapid, alternating movements across a joint associated with increased muscular tone and hyperactive reflexes.

Conduit d'approche: The tendency of certain aphasic patients to approach the correct production of a target word through a series of successive phonemic alterations.

Conduit d'ecart: The tendency of certain aphasic patients to move away from the target word through the production of a series of successive phonemic alterations.

Confabulation: An involuntary tendency to fill in gaps in memory with fabricated information, usually seen in patients with amnestic syndromes.

Cortical deafness: The inability to hear as a result of cerebral lesions in the central auditory pathways.

Crossed aphasia: Aphasia resulting from a lesion to the right hemisphere in right-handers.

Diplopia: Double vision.

Dysdiadochokinesia: A breakdown in the fluidity of movement usually associated with cerebellar dysfunction, often measured by tests of rapid alternating movements.

Dysmetria: The impaired guidance of movement to a target, resulting in under- or overshooting.

Dysphagia: A disorder of swallowing.

Dystonia: An abnormality of muscle tone.

Echolalia: Involuntary repetition of someone else's words.

Edema: Swelling of tissue due to excess fluid within the tissue.

Encephalitis: Inflammation of the brain, usually of infectious origin.

Fasciculation: Ripple-like contractions of small groups of muscles seen, for example, in amyotropic lateral sclerosis.

Gegenhalten: Abnormality of muscle tone characterized by progressively increasing resistance to passive movement.

Horner's syndrome: Ptosis (drooping of the upper eyelid), meiosis (constriction of the pupil), and anhydrosis (dryness of the skin) on one side of the face, associated with sympathetic nerve damage.

Hyperesthesia: A pathological increase in sensation.

Hyperpathia: A pathological increase in pain sensation.

Intention tremor: A tremor that increases in amplitude with voluntary movement.

Limbic system: Phylogenetically old anatomical structures (e.g., hippocampus, amygdala, septal nuclei) that are located deep within the cerebral hemisphere and contribute to emotional behavior.

Logorrhea: Excessive speech output.

Meningitis: Inflammation of the meninges (membranes covering the brain), usually of infectious origin.

Meningioma: A slowly growing brain tumor of meningeal origin.

Micrographia: Small, often illegible, handwriting usually associated with basal ganglia dysfunction.

Mnestic: Pertaining to memory.

Myoclonus: Sudden, rapid, involuntary contraction of a muscle or of muscle groups.

Neoplasm: Tumor, or new growth, that may be benign or malignant.

Nocturia: Nighttime urinary incontinence.

Nystagmus: Instability of gaze fixation manifested by rhythmic jiggling of the eyes in any direction.

Palilalia: Involuntary repetition of one's own words or phrases uttered with increasing rapidity and decreasing clarity and volume. Usually associated with basal ganglia disease.

Pronator drift: The tendency of the extended arm to turn inward, usually secondary to pyramidal system damage.

Prosopagnosia: Failure to recognize familiar faces, usually resulting from bilateral occipitotemporal lesions.

Proprioception: Awareness of the position of a limb in space.

Pure word deafness: A rare syndrome in which the patient can hear but cannot process speech sounds for meaning, although his or her own spontaneous speech, reading, and writing skills are intact.

Romberg's sign: Failure to maintain a steady, standing balance with eyes closed.

Scotoma: A blind spot.

Sinistrality: Left-handedness.

Simultanagnosia: The inability to identify the totality of a visual scene despite the ability to identify the separate components, usually associated with bilateral occipitoparietal lesions.

Split brain: A condition in which the corpus callosum has been divided, so that the transfer of the information between the two cerebral hemispheres is reduced.

Status epilepticus: A condition in which epileptic attacks succeed each other so rapidly that the patient does not regain consciousness between the attacks.

Stenosis: Narrowing or constriction of a tubular opening such as a blood vessel.

Subluxation: A condition of separation of dislocation of a body part, often occurring in the shoulder joint of a paralyzed arm.

Syncope: Fainting.

Tinnitus: Ringing in the ears.

Todd's paralysis: Transient suppression of neural function following epileptic seizure, sometimes resulting in hemiparesis and speech disturbance.

Tachistoscope: An apparatus for presenting visual stimuli in a controlled, rapid fashion. May be used to test lateralized cerebral functions.

Utilization behavior: An involuntary drive to manipulate objects in the environment despite instructions to refrain. Associated with frontal lobe disease.

Vertebro-basilar insufficiency: A transient decrease in cerebral oxygenation caused by stenosis of the vertebral and basilar arteries.

Wada test: Injection of sodium amytal into the carotid artery resulting in transient suppression of the functions of the ipsilateral cerebral hemisphere.

Xanthochromia: A pinkish-yellow discoloration of cerebrospinal fluid indicating bleeding into the subarachnoid space.

II. Acronyms

A.D.: Right ear.

ADL's: Activities of daily living.

A FIB: Atrial fibrilation.

AKA: Above the knee amputation.

ARF: Acute renal failure.

ASA: Aspirin.

A.S.: Left ear.

A.U.: Both ears.

AVM: Arteriovenous malformation.

BAER: Brainstem auditory evoked response.

BP: Blood pressure.

B.I.D.: Twice a day.

BUN: Blood urea nitrogen.

DVT: Deep vein thrombosis.

CABG: Coronary artery bypass graft.

CAD: Coronary artery disease.

CHF: Congestive heart failure.

CHI: Closed head injury.
CNS: Central nervous system.
COPD: Chronic obstructive pulmonary disease.
CSF: Cerebrospinal fluid.
CT: Computerized tomography.
CVD: Cardiovascular disease.
DM: Diabetes mellitus.
DNR: Do not resuscitate.
DOB: Date of birth.
DSS: Double simultaneous stimulation.
ECG: Electrocardiogram.
ECT: Electroconvulsive (shock) therapy.
EEG: Electroencephalogram.
EKG: Electrocardiogram.
EMG: Electromyography.
ENG: Electronystagmography.
EOM: Extraocular movements.
ER: Emergency room.
ETOH: Alcohol.
FBS: Fasting blood sugar.
FFM: Fine finger movement.
FH: Family history.
FIRDA: Frontal intermittent rhythmic delta activity.
FUO: Fever of unknown origin.
GI: Gastrointestinal.
GSW: Gunshot wound.
HA: Headaches.
HCTZ: Hydrochlorothiazide.
HEENT: Head, eyes, ears, nose, and throat.
HTN: Hypertension.
ICA: Internal carotid artery.
IDDM: Insulin dependent diabetes mellitus.
IVA: Inferior vena cava.
LOC: Loss of consciousness.
LOS: Length of stay.
LLE: Left lower extremity.
LP: Lumbar puncture.
LUE: Left upper extremity.
MCA: Middle cerebral artery.
MRI: Magnetic resonance imaging.
MS: Mental status.
MVA: Motor vehicle accident.
NAD: No acute distress.

NIIDS: Non-insulin dependent diabetes.
NL: Normal.
NPH: Normal pressure hydrocephalus.
NSAID: Nonsteroidal anti-inflammatory drug.
O.D.: Right eye.
O.R.: Operating room.
O.S.: Left eye.
O.U.: Both eyes.
PERRLA: Pupils equal, round, reactive to light and accommodation.
PET: Positron emission tomography.
PTA: Prior to admission.
PUD: Peptic ulcer disease.
Q.I.D.: Four times a day.
RAM: Rapid alternating movements.
RBC: Red blood count.
RIND: Reversible ischemic neurological disease.
RLE: Right lower extremity.
RLQ: Right lower quadrant.
ROM: Range of motion.
RUE: Right upper extremity.
SOB: Shortness of breath.
S/P: Status post.
SPEP: Serum protein electrophoresis.
SSEP: Somatosensory evoked potentials.
TIA: Transient ischemic attack.
TLE: Temporal lobe epilepsy.
TURP: Transurethral resection of prostate.
UGI: Upper gastrointestinal.
UTI: Urinary tract infection.
VFD: Visual field defect.
VSS: Vital signs stable.
WDWN: Well developed, well nourished.
WNL: Within normal limits.

Index

agrammatism, 166, 171, 219–220, 222
agraphia, 21
AIDS virus, 49
alcohol use, 50
Alzheimer's disease, 26, 28, 78–79, 80, 92, 261
Alzheimer's Disease and Related Disorders Association, 262
American Speech, Hearing, and Language Association, 261
aneurysm, 63, 67, 71
anger, 257
anomia, 25, 36, 77, 79
anxiety, 56, 246, 257
aphasia
  classification of (cortical vs. subcortical, fluent vs. nonfluent), 35, 38, 39, 41, 42, 44, 45, 105, 106, 119
  family issues in, 159–160, 197–198, 227, 256, 257–258, 261, 262
  legal implications of, 259–261
  neurobehavioral aspects of, 253
  neuropsychiatric aspects of, 254–256
  psychosocial aspects of, 256–258, 261–262
  relative impairment vs. relative preservation in, 113
aphasia, anomic
  after head injury, 70
  and Alzheimer's disease, 79
  and hypomania, 255–256
  auditory comprehension in, 39
  differential diagnosis of, 35–41
  lesion sites in, 25, 76

  repetition skills in, 41
  sample responses of, 151, 152
  speech samples, 108, 111
  test performance in, 100
aphasia, anterior capsular/putaminal
  candidacy for Helm Elicited Program for Syntax Stimulation in, 222
  differential diagnosis of, 35, 41–45
  in dementia, 79
  lesion site in, 43
aphasia, Broca's
  auditory comprehension in, 39
  candidacy for Helm Elicited Program for Syntax Stimulation in, 222
  course of therapy in, 239
  differential diagnosis of, 35–41
  Index of Grammatical Support in, 168
  lesion sites in, 21–23, 30
  narrative writing in, 129
  repetition skills in, 41
  sample Communicative Effectiveness Profile for, 170
  sample picture descriptions pre/post treatment for, 171–173
  sample responses of, 147, 152
  speech samples for, 108, 109, 219
  test performance in, 100
aphasia, conduction
  auditory comprehension in, 39
  differential diagnosis of, 35–41
  emotional reactions in, 256
  lesion sites in, 23–25, 30, 256
  narrative writing in, 128

About the Authors

Nancy Helm-Estabrooks, Sc.D., Professor of Neurology (Speech Pathology) at Boston University School of Medicine, is a Senior Research Investigator at Boston University's Aphasia Research Center at the Boston Veterans Administration Medical Center, and a Core Faculty Member at the Boston University Graduate School Division of Medical and Dental Sciences. She has authored numerous tests, books, chapters, and journal articles, particularly in the area of aphasia diagnosis and rehabilitation.

Martin L. Albert, M.D., Professor of Neurology at Boston University School of Medicine, is Director of Behavioral Neurosciences at the Boston Veterans Administration Medical Center and is Co-Principal Investigator of the Boston University Aphasia Research Center. He has authored or co-authored more than 100 books and articles in behavioral neuroscience, with an emphasis on aphasia, aging, and dementia.